VEGAN
BASICS

INCLUDES 50+ RECIPES

Your Guide to the Essentials of a Plant-Based Diet—and How It Can Work for You!

**VEGAN
GUIDELINES**

**STARTER
RECIPES**

**LIFESTYLE
ADJUSTMENTS**

Adams Media
New York London Toronto Sydney New Delhi

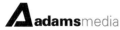

Adams Media
An Imprint of Simon & Schuster, Inc.
57 Littlefield Street
Avon, Massachusetts 02322

First Adams Media trade paperback edition January 2019

ADAMS MEDIA and colophon are trademarks of Simon & Schuster.

For information about special discounts for bulk purchases, please contact Simon & Schuster Special Sales at 1-866-506-1949 or business@simonandschuster.com.

The Simon & Schuster Speakers Bureau can bring authors to your live event. For more information or to book an event contact the Simon & Schuster Speakers Bureau at 1-866-248-3049 or visit our website at www.simonspeakers.com.

Interior design by Stephanie Hannus
Interior images © 123RF; Getty Images

Manufactured in the United States of America

10 9 8 7 6 5 4 3 2 1

Library of Congress Cataloging-in-Publication Data has been applied for.

ISBN 978-1-5072-1013-0
ISBN 978-1-5072-1014-7 (ebook)

Many of the designations used by manufacturers and sellers to distinguish their products are claimed as trademarks. Where those designations appear in this book and Simon & Schuster, Inc., was aware of a trademark claim, the designations have been printed with initial capital letters.

The information in this book should not be used for diagnosing or treating any health problem. Not all diet and exercise plans suit everyone.

You should always consult a trained medical professional before starting a diet, taking any form of medication, or embarking on any fitness or weight-training program. The author and publisher disclaim any liability arising directly or indirectly from the use of this book.

Always follow safety and commonsense cooking protocols while using kitchen utensils, operating ovens and stoves, and handling uncooked food. If children are assisting in the preparation of any recipe, they should always be supervised by an adult.

Contains material adapted from the following titles published by Adams Media, an Imprint of Simon & Schuster, Inc.: *The Everything® Vegan Cookbook* by Jolinda Hackett with Lorena Novak Bull, copyright © 2010, ISBN 978-1-4405-0216-3; *The Everything® Guide to Being Vegetarian* by Alexandra Greeley, copyright © 2009, ISBN 978-1-60550-051-5; *The Everything® Vegan Pregnancy Book* by Reed Mangels, PhD, RD, LD, FADA, copyright © 2011, ISBN 978-1-4405-2551-3; *The Daily Vegan Planner* by Jolinda Hackett with Nicole Cormier, copyright © 2012, ISBN 978-1-4405-2998-6; *The Everything® Guide to Nutrition* by Nicole Cormier, RD, LDN, copyright © 2011, ISBN 978-1-4405-1030–4; *The Everything® Vegan Baking Cookbook* by Lorena Novak Bull, RD, copyright © 2012, ISBN 978-1-4405-2997-9; *The Everything® Vegan Paleo Cookbook* by Daelyn Fortney, copyright © 2015, ISBN 978-1-4405-9022-1.

Contents

3: Plant Protein Is Your Friend 73

4: Benefits, Risks, and Concerns of the Vegan Diet 89

5: Ingredients for Healthy Vegan Cooking 111

Introduction

You've heard a lot about the benefits of going vegan. It lowers cholesterol levels, reduces your risk of heart disease, helps you to lose weight, and so much more. But with so many rules and restrictions, where do you begin?

With the basics.

Vegan Basics teaches you everything you need to know about the vegan diet in a quick, easy-to-understand way. Wondering what you can eat? You'll discover the wide variety of delicious foods included in the vegan diet. Confused about what makes a food vegan? You'll find a clear explanation along with easy-to-follow guidelines. Worried an all-plant diet will leave you feeling hungry all the time? Not a problem! You'll learn about the many filling foods you can enjoy and find tips for beating cravings. Plus, there are more than fifty recipes so delicious, you won't believe they're vegan!

You'll learn the ins and outs of plant-based eating. How you apply the information is up to you. Maybe you want to increase the amount of fruits and veggies in your diet, or maybe you're looking for a healthy alternative to red meat and cheese, or maybe you're concerned about animals and the environment. Whatever your motives, with the *Vegan Basics* covered, you can be confident and successful in your diet decisions.

No matter what your reasons are for trying plant-based eating, this book is here to help you understand the vegan diet and apply it to your life—easily and effectively.

1

Getting Started on the Vegan Diet

This chapter will give you an overview of the vegan diet and introduce you to the wide variety of plant-based foods available to you.

Vegans can eat anything but choose not to eat certain foods. When thinking about what to include and exclude in your diet, consider your reasons and values for choosing a vegan diet. Does eating a particular food align or conflict with these values? Whatever your diet may be, stick with your personal values and goals rather than dictionary definitions.

Plant-Based Diets

Eating plants as food is basic to all vegetarians, but over time people have devised many different vegetarian categories to suit their various beliefs and lifestyles. For beginners, the distinctions may seem bewildering.

Lacto-Ovo: Perhaps the largest group, these vegetarians eat both dairy products and eggs, but no meat of any kind. Their food plan is broad and offers substantial choices to include greens, grains, fruits, and legumes, plus moderate amounts of nuts, dairy products, eggs, and plant oils, and in the smallest quantities, sweets.

Lacto: This group omits eggs but does include all dairy products in a diet that otherwise resembles the lacto-ovo food plan.

Ovo: These vegetarians include eggs but omit all dairy products in a diet that otherwise resembles the typical vegetarian one.

Vegan: Following the strictest plant-based diet, a vegan excludes eating or using all animal meats or products, including all dairy, eggs, and honey. And a strict vegan will not wear anything made from silk, leather, or wool. They are careful to avoid eating any processed foods that may have required animal products in their manufacture, such as refined sugar. While the eating plan sounds restrictive, careful vegans plan their meals to include a wide range of nutrient-dense foods.

Flexitarian: Whether you call this group flexitarian or semivegetarian, these people do include some meat in their diet. Some people may eat fish (pescatarian) but no red meat or poultry; for health reasons, this particular form of vegetarianism is increasingly popular. Some may eat poultry, but no red meat or fish. And others may limit their meat intake to an occasional meal. But to the active vegetarian community, flexitarians are just vegetarians in the making.

Veganism

Vegan is a word used to explain a complete lifestyle, one that is lived in a manner that avoids as much harm to sentient beings as possible. Ethical vegans not only shun all animal products in food; they also eliminate the use of animal-sourced items in their overall day-to-day lives.

The Vegan Society, formed in 1944 and based in the United Kingdom, defines *veganism* as "a way of living that seeks to exclude, as far as possible and practicable, all forms of exploitation of, and cruelty to, animals for food, clothing, and any other purpose." The Vegetarian Resource Group, a nonprofit educational group in the United States, says, "Vegetarians do not eat meat, fish, or poultry. Vegans, in addition to being vegetarian, do not use other animal products and by-products such as eggs, dairy products, honey, leather, fur, silk, wool, cosmetics, and soaps derived from animal products."

Foods to Avoid

The vegan diet encompasses a vegetarian diet—so all meats, fish, and poultry are excluded—and extends to exclude any animal product or by-product—including eggs, milk, cheese and other dairy products, and honey.

Vegans also try to avoid foods that may have used animal products in their production. Some ingredients derived from animal products may be fairly obvious, such as chicken or beef broth or casein from milk. Other ingredients may be less apparent. Gelatin, for example, is derived from animal bones and connective tissue. Carmine (sometimes called cochineal) is a red food coloring derived from the dried bodies of female cochineal insects. Some sugar companies process sugar through a bone char in order to remove color from the sugar. Wine production may also involve animal products. Clarifying agents for wine include egg whites, casein (from milk), gelatin, and isinglass (from fish). Foods fortified with vitamin D contain one of two forms of vitamin D, D_2, or D_3. Vitamin D_3 is typically made from lanolin, an oily substance from sheep's wool.

In order to make decisions about which products or ingredients fit into your values scheme as you follow a vegan diet, be sure to read ingredient listings on products.

Guidelines for Vegan Foods

Determining whether an item is vegan is actually quite simple. Ask yourself, "Did this come from a living creature?" If the answer is yes, then it isn't vegan.

- What about seafood? Does seafood come from a living creature? Fish, lobsters, and shrimp are all living creatures; therefore, seafood is not vegan.
- What about honey? Does honey come from a living creature? Honey is made by honeybees, which are living creatures; therefore, honey is not vegan.
- What about gelatin? Does gelatin come from a living creature? Gelatin is obtained through the boiling of bones, ligaments, and skin of animals; therefore, gelatin is not vegan.

In short, anything that is derived from an animal is off-limits in the vegan diet.

Of course, it's easy to know not to consume a hamburger, macaroni and cheese, or an omelet, and it's just as easy to know that salads, spaghetti with marinara, and tofu over rice are all on the "Yes" list, but things get tricky when trying to indulge in convenient foods—boxed, canned, and prepackaged meals. Reading food labels is imperative when practicing a vegan lifestyle. However, in reality, even those who do not have dietary restrictions should adopt the habit of reading labels. It's important to know what's going into your body.

Food to Eat

Vegans eat a wide variety of foods, many of which are familiar to those eating a more traditional American diet. For example, a vegan breakfast could include orange juice, toast with jelly, oatmeal with raisins, and coffee or tea. Lunch could be a standard PB and J sandwich with an apple and some chips, while dinner could be bean burritos, a tossed salad with Italian dressing, and apple crisp.

Vegans may also choose some foods that can seem less familiar. For instance, breakfast could include vegan "sausage" and pancakes, lunch could feature a veggie burger or dog, and dinner could be barbecued seitan over quinoa with vegan biscuits and a frozen dessert based on coconut milk.

Many foods traditionally made with animal products are available in vegan form in large supermarkets or natural foods stores. From macaroni and cheese to fish sticks to barbecue ribs, there are convenient vegan options.

Vegan cookbooks and websites offer recipes for making your favorite foods vegan. Recipes can include simple tricks like replacing eggs with flaxseed or tofu, or they may feature more complicated formulas to make dishes that taste like seafood or dairy-based cheese.

Many restaurants have vegan options on their menus. If you don't see something that you like, don't hesitate to ask. Here are a few ideas:

- Veggie no-cheese pizza (ask if the dough contains cheese, milk, or eggs)
- Moo Shu vegetables (ask your server to tell the kitchen to leave out eggs)
- Falafel
- Indian curries and dal (ask for them to be made with oil instead of ghee (clarified butter)
- Bean burritos and tacos (hold the cheese and sour cream; check for lard in refried beans)

Meat Substitutes

These days you can find a vegan version of almost any meat or seafood product. These "not meats" are often made from soy or seitan, although other beans and grains are sometimes used, especially in veggie burgers. Check labels—some have eggs, egg whites, or cheese added. From Thanksgiving unturkey to Fourth of July veggie dogs, there are products for every occasion. You can find soy "sausages," made from soy proteins, as links or as a compact product packed in a tube. In the tube, the soy meat is easy to crumble and sauté like its pork sausage counterpart; alternatively, it slices easily and panfries like a patty.

These products are often high in protein and may be fortified with iron, zinc, or vitamin B_{12}. The downside is that they tend to be expensive.

Tempeh

Tempeh has a crumbly texture that some find reminds them of meat. It originated in Indonesia and is made from whole soybeans that have been fermented, either alone or with a grain. It needs steaming, simmering, or frying before eating. Look for tempeh in the refrigerator section of natural foods stores. Several different kinds are usually available, but they're all interchangeable.

Tempeh is a popular addition to soups and casseroles. Most tempeh recipes will turn out better if your tempeh is simmered in a bit of water or vegetable broth first. This improves the digestibility of the tempeh, softens it up, and decreases the cooking time. And if you add some seasonings such as soy sauce, garlic powder, or some herbs, it will increase the flavor as well.

TVP

TVP (textured vegetable protein) is made from soy flour. TVP is inexpensive and has such a meaty texture that many budget-conscious nonvegetarian cooks use it to stretch their dollar, adding it to homemade burgers and meatloaf.

It is often found in the bulk section of natural foods stores. TVP is sold in chunks and granules and may be flavored to taste like beef or chicken. For the best deal, buy it in bulk. TVP is usually found in small crumbles, but some specialty shops also sell it in strips or chunks.

TVP must be soaked in boiling water to rehydrate it. It can then be used in chili, sloppy joes, spaghetti sauce, and other recipes in place of ground beef.

Seitan

If you've eaten in a vegetarian Chinese restaurant, you've probably eaten seitan. Seitan is made from gluten, the protein part of wheat. It has a chewy texture and can be baked, boiled, or stir-fried. Seitan is also called wheat meat and can be found in the refrigerated section of natural foods stores. You can also make your own seitan; a gluten flour mix makes it easy. Shop for vital wheat gluten, also called wheat gluten flour, at your natural foods store in the bulk section or baking aisle.

Seitan expands when it cooks, so use more broth and a larger pot than you think you might need, and add an extra bouillon cube for maximum flavor if you like.

Tofu

Unflavored soy milk is mixed with a coagulant to make tofu in a process that is similar to making cheese. It's a minimally processed, low-fat source of calcium and protein. Plain tofu comes in either firm, extra-firm, or silken (also called silk or soft tofu), and many grocers stock a variety of prebaked or flavored tofu.

For best results, choose the right kind of tofu for the dish you'll be using it in. Silken tofu (often available in shelf-stable packaging) is best used for dishes where you want a creamy consistency—shakes, puddings, salad dressings, sauces, and pie fillings.

Firm or extra-firm tofu is a better choice for stir-fries and other dishes where you want the tofu to keep its shape.

Once a package of refrigerated tofu is opened, any unused tofu should be refrigerated and covered with water. Shelf-stable tofu should be refrigerated after opening but does not need to be covered with water.

Plant "Milks"

Soy milk is made by soaking, grinding, and straining soybeans. It is available in both shelf-stable and refrigerated forms and comes in flavors like vanilla, chocolate, and carob. In mid-December, you can often find eggnog-flavored soy milk. Vegans often rely on fortified soy milk as a source of calcium, vitamin B_{12}, and vitamin D, so check the label of the brand you prefer to make sure these important nutrients have been added.

In addition to soy milk, many other plant milks are available based on hemp seeds, almonds, oats, rice, and coconut. Which to choose is a personal preference, although if you are relying on plant milks as sources of key nutrients, be aware that not all are fortified and check the label to find one that meets your needs. Soy milk is highest in protein with 6–10 grams of protein in a cup. Oat milk and hemp milk have about half as much protein; and rice, coconut, and almond milks only provide about 1 gram of protein per cup. Unflavored, original, or plain varieties of plant milks work best in savory dishes. Flavored milks (vanilla, chocolate, carob, and others) are sweeter and work in desserts and drinks.

Vegan "Cheeses" and "Yogurts"

Vegan cheese is typically made from rice, soybeans, peas, or nuts. It can be used in recipes that call for dairy cheese but does not have the same nutritional profile. Some brands of vegan cheese do have calcium added. Most are quite low in protein. Grating or shredding vegan cheese helps it melt and combine with other ingredients.

Packages of nondairy products that say "lactose-free" but do not say "vegan" or "casein-free" frequently contain casein, a protein that comes from cow's milk. Casein is what gives cheese its stretchy quality when melted. Cheese that contains casein is not vegan. Some brands of vegan cheese use other ingredients to mimic casein's stretchiness.

Vegan yogurt can be found in the dairy case of supermarkets and natural foods stores. Yogurt is commonly made from soy milk; coconut milk-based yogurt is a recent addition. Several brands of vegan yogurt are fortified with vitamins and minerals to resemble dairy yogurt.

Dairy in Soy Cheeses

Many nondairy products do actually contain dairy, even if it says "nondairy" right there on the package! Nondairy creamer and soy cheeses are notorious for this. Look for casein or whey on the ingredients list, particularly if you suffer from dairy allergies, and, if you're allergic to soy, look for nut- or rice-based vegan cheeses.

Not All Vegan Foods Are Healthy

Just because a food (or recipe) is vegan doesn't mean it's healthy! If health is your main concern for going vegan, you may do well to avoid vegan cream cheese. Vegan cream cheese usually contains hydrogenated oils, which are admittedly nearly as bad for your system as red meat. Nonhydrogenated vegan cream cheese is available, but unfortunately, it just doesn't taste as good!

Nutritional Yeast

Nutritional yeast is used in vegan recipes to add a cheese flavor. It can be sprinkled on popcorn or vegetables. Watch out for brewer's yeast, which many well-meaning people insist is the same as nutritional yeast. It's not. Brewer's yeast has a bitter flavor. You'll know it's nutritional yeast if you see pale yellow flakes or granules. Depending on where you live, nutritional yeast may be called "savory yeast flakes" or "nutritional food yeast."

Nutritional yeast containing B_{12} is commonly available in packages and in bulk food bins. Check the label to make sure the product you are using contains it.

Egg Replacers

Because you can chop, scramble, whip, or beat it, and it adds both texture and protein, tofu is an excellent egg substitute. Commercial egg replacers containing various binding agents are often used to replace eggs in vegan baking. You can find powdered egg replacers at health-food stores and many whole-food markets; to use them properly, follow package directions. But remember, egg replacers and egg substitutes do not cook up the same way eggs do, so you may have to experiment to get the results you are looking for.

See Chapter 5 for a variety of egg substitute recipes that can be used in baking.

Ground flaxseeds can be blended with water and used as egg replacers. A tablespoon and a half of ground flaxseeds blended with ¼ cup of water can substitute for a large egg. You can purchase whole flaxseeds and grind them yourself or purchase them already ground (flaxseed meal). Opened packages of flaxseed should be stored in the freezer.

Leafy Greens

According to the United States Department of Agriculture (USDA), *leafy greens* refers to such obvious candidates as lettuce, cabbage, chard, collards, kale, and spinach, but the category also includes broccoli—and all are members of the Brassicaceae family with valuable cancer-fighting phytochemicals. As members of the crucifer family, the leafy greens contain cancer-fighting phytochemicals known as isothiocyanates. But scientists warn that food-borne illnesses from improperly handled greens have also risen, which means consumers must be especially careful of how they handle their produce.

Greens are easy to cook. They are extremely versatile and work as well in salads and sandwiches as in stir-fries and stews, and they have flavor profiles from pleasantly bland to sharp and biting.

Popular greens include arugula, collard greens, kale, mustard greens, Swiss chard, and turnip greens.

Asian Greens

Thanks to the growth spurt in Asian restaurants and Asian markets in the United States, an increasing number of Americans can identify and feel comfortable with cooking and eating Asian vegetables, particularly leafy Asian greens. As members of the cruciferous vegetable family, Asian greens add both nutrients and interesting flavors to your family meals. And, in general, these greens are easy to work with and cook up quickly for a range of tasty dishes; some are tender enough to toss into the salad bowl without any precooking.

Bok choy, Napa cabbage, choy sum, and Chinese broccoli are all examples of Asian greens.

Many Asian vegetables have more than one scientific name and several different marketplace titles. For example, bok choy is also named pak choi; the long, white Chinese cabbage is commonly tagged Napa cabbage; and choy sum is also known as yu choy and may be spelled choi sam. Chinese broccoli is also known as gai lan, kai laan, or Chinese kale. And to mix it all up, many grocers use the general term *Chinese cabbage* to refer to numerous cruciferous Chinese greens.

Sturdy Greens

Among the members of the vegetable kingdom, a small group of sturdy greens needs the tenderizing effect of the cookpot to make them palatable and edible. But once cooked and ready for the plate, these veggies contribute both taste and some gastronomic diversions for the vegetarian—or for anyone. These vegetables include the artichoke; broccoli and the Italian broccoli rabe (no relation); and Brussels sprouts, a mini cabbagelike green that most people love to hate.

According to the USDA, 1 cup of chopped raw broccoli contains 31 calories, 2.4 grams total fiber, 43 grams of calcium, 81 grams of vitamin C, and 288 grams of potassium.

Lettuces

The array of true lettuce varieties in the produce section and at farmers' markets has exploded, from the time-honored iceberg heads and romaine to Bibb, Boston, Ruby (or red leaf), chicory, corn salad, oak leaf, Buttercrunch, and Black Seeded Simpson, plus dozens and dozens more. According to the Centers for Disease Control and Prevention (CDC), all these varieties fall into one of the four main categories: crisphead, butterhead, loose-leaf, and cos or romaine.

Most lettuce leaves, while not nutrient powerhouses, do convey some essential vitamins and that all-important fiber all people need. Besides, for folks on a diet, few foods contain fewer calories, ounce for ounce, and lettuce has no fat or cholesterol. For example, 1 cup of chopped raw romaine lettuce contains 10 calories and 0 grams of fat, cholesterol, and sodium. Both the calories and fat come with what you put into the salad bowl to keep the lettuce company.

Experts point out the lettuce leaves—particularly those that are darker green—do contain such vitamins as A and C and offer calcium, potassium, and beta-carotene. Plus, lettuce leaves are a good source for those all-important phytonutrients that work as antioxidants to fight illness. Even the iceberg lettuce, so often spurned by salad enthusiasts as being a tasteless second-best, has not only made a glamorous salad bowl comeback; it also contains some vitamin A. Note that nutrient values also vary by lettuce type.

Vegetables

Tomatoes, corn, asparagus, peas, peppers, cucumbers, green beans, and chilies: these assorted vegetables are so familiar in the kitchen that few cooks need an introduction. And most grow easily in a garden plot with enough room to accommodate their spreading vines and leafing stalks. Seeds and edible pods—from green beans to corn on the cob—are sweet when young and best if cooked straight from the garden or field. In the market, avoid any that look wrinkled or yellowing, which means they are old.

The summertime favorites—tomatoes, peppers, cucumbers, eggplants, and chilies—are basically available year-round, but as any cook knows, their flavors reach their peak in the warm summer months. At home, most work well in a variety of recipes, making them ready nutrient sources.

Fruits

In the kitchen, ripe fruits of any classification can come to the rescue morning, noon, and night—and in between. Fruits can stand alone and be enjoyed raw, with maybe a drizzle of agave nectar, a pinch of salt, or added to a salad. On the other hand, many fruits cook up well in syrups, pies, cakes, jams, pancakes, waffles, soufflés, dairy-free ice cream, and puddings, and they can accent savory entrées with just a hint of sweetness to tempt the palate: plantains with black beans is one such example.

Fruits are healthful props for the modern diet. As the USDA points out, fruit—and vegetable—consumption may lower the risk factors for several chronic diseases, such as heart disease, type 2 diabetes, certain cancers, development of kidney stones, and, of course, obesity.

The USDA further details those nutrients in most fruits that act as health-promoting agents: potassium, in bananas, cantaloupe, and orange juice, for example, for possibly normalizing blood pressure; vitamin C for tissue growth and repair; folate for red blood cell formation; and that all-important fiber, for keeping the intestines functioning properly and for possibly reducing levels of blood cholesterol.

Experts from the Harvard School of Public Health say you should eat about 2 cups of fruit a day to promote, among other health benefits, better eyesight.

Mushrooms

Versatile and nutritious—and low in calories—mushrooms can be puréed into creamy soups, rolled into burritos, and tossed into salads. According to the USDA, mushrooms are sources of copper, potassium, and folate, to name a few nutrients. Asian studies of mushrooms suggest that mushrooms may help boost the immune system and may contain valuable antioxidants.

Years ago, the only mushroom readily available was the white variety, and that was often sold canned rather than fresh. Today's markets, however, offer consumers many of the thousands of wild and cultivated mushroom varieties. Look for such mushrooms as chanterelle, oyster, shiitake, enoki, portobello, cremini, maitake, and the very pricey morel at your market. In your Asian market, look for several dried varieties, such as the shiitake and the straw mushrooms.

Besides the popular white or button mushrooms, the very versatile portobello mushroom may be the consumer's top pick. Not only is the portobello a fine protein source, its dense, chewy texture makes for pleasurable eating. Because its cap may be large enough to replace a slice of bread, the portobello makes a delicious sandwich, and it can be grilled, roasted, stir-fried, and eaten raw.

Roots and Tubers

Plentiful and easy on the budget, root and tuberous vegetables—from potatoes to beets to parsnips to sunchokes—fill many of the bins in the supermarket year-round. Many, like the potato and sweet potato, are so popular that they turn up often on the dinner plate—and that's a bonus for vegans and nonvegans alike: roots and tubers generally offer few calories, no fat, some fiber, but many nutrients, depending on the vegetable.

Potatoes do supply some nutrients and fiber if you eat the potato skin. But while potatoes—which now come in numerous shapes and colors, some as small as thimbles and others darkly purple—are undeniably delicious, they are also an easily digested starch that may result in a rapid rise in blood sugar. According to the Harvard School of Public Health, potatoes and refined carbohydrates may play a role in the onset of type 2 diabetes. So, while you may love potatoes, you should eat potatoes sparingly, and more often substitute the sweet for the white potato.

Grains

As a food group, grains include oats, barley, wheat, rye, brown rice, amaranth, buckwheat, millet, quinoa, and sorghum. All these grains—some are "pseudograins"—are eaten whole or processed into the various cereals, pastas, tortillas, and breads you eat. A pseudograin is a seed or kernel that is not a member of the grass family but is treated like a grain in the kitchen. According to the Wheat Foods Council, these include amaranth, flaxseed, quinoa, and buckwheat.

Grain products are divided into two categories: refined and whole grain. Food manufacturers refine whole grains by milling them and removing the bran, the endosperm, and the germ of the grain. Refining does yield a product with a finer texture and a longer shelf life, but during the milling process, many of the whole grains' nutrients and fiber are discarded.

After processing, manufacturers enrich the refined product by adding back some vitamins and iron, but the end result does not compare nutritionally to the original whole grains. You will find many refined grains products in the marketplace, including flours, cereals, and pastas.

Whole grains are just that: whole, with the bran, germ, and endosperm intact. Examples include brown rice, whole-wheat flour, oats, and corn and whole cornmeal.

Rice

Rice is grown almost everywhere in the world, and it is truly a beloved food for numerous reasons: it is plentiful, delicious, inexpensive, and very filling.

Rice is also nutritious and contains several vitamins and minerals, complex carbohydrates, and no fat. Because it still contains the bran, brown rice provides more nutrients and has a more complex, slightly nutty taste.

Rice is generally divided into three categories: long grain, medium grain, and short grain. And within those categories, you'll find numerous varieties, from the long-grain fragrant basmati and jasmine rice preferred in India and parts of Asia to the regular unscented long-grain rice the Chinese and Americans cook. Medium- and short-grain rice tends to be moister and plumper—and the very short-grain rice used for sushi has a sticky quality that lets the grains cling together.

Nut and Seed Butters

Nut and seed butters add protein, calories, and essential fats to vegan diets. Well-stocked stores feature almond butter, hazelnut butter, cashew butter, macadamia butter, and more. They can be used for sandwiches, to add richness to a smoothie, or to flavor soups, stews, and grain dishes. For those with nut allergies, try soy nut butter (made from roasted soybeans), sunflower seed butter, and tahini (sesame seed butter). Even if you still prefer peanut butter, check out some of the flavored peanut butters—from spicy to cinnamon-raisin.

Beans, Nuts, Lentils, and Chickpeas

For vegans, such protein powerhouses as legumes—beans and lentils—and nuts are the foundation of an all-veg menu, for these foods not only contain protein, good carbs, fiber, and micronutrients; they also, in the case of nuts, add some good-for-you fats. And for ease of cooking, these can't be beat. Almost every legume comes precooked in a can, and nuts are sold roasted and shelled ready for the breakfast, lunch, or dinner plate.

Most supermarkets carry the common brown lentils, but for real gastronomic explorations, you should try the tiny French green lentils and the Italian black lentils, or take a trip to an Indian grocer, whose shelves will display a variety of lentil shapes and colors. You'll find whole or split lentils and even some lentils with the hulls removed.

Vegan Sweets

Vegans with a sweet tooth can find all sorts of vegan chocolates, baked goods, and frozen desserts at vegan bakeries or candy stores, natural foods stores, and online. It's also easy to make your own desserts, and you'll find some dessert recipes later in this book.

If you have a favorite recipe that calls for honey, or if you like something sweet to add to herbal tea, you might try agave nectar. Agave nectar is a liquid sweetener produced from the juice of a succulent plant. Agave nectar mainly provides sugar and calories, so it should be used in moderation.

The Food and Drug Administration (FDA) has approved four sugar substitutes, or sweeteners, that are safe—and sweet—and currently on the market. These include saccharin, aspartame, sucralose (sold as the product Splenda), and acesulfame potassium. If taken in moderate amounts, none pose health risks, not even saccharin, once thought to be linked to certain cancers.

Starting a Vegan Diet

Common advice when going vegan is to eliminate red meats followed by white meats, and then spend some time eating just fish or a vegetarian diet before eliminating eggs, dairy, and other trace ingredients. While this method intuitively seems like a good idea and indeed works for some people, it's also a little bit backward. Here's why. Dairy, and cheese in particular, is often the most difficult food to eliminate from your diet. This is a good argument for gradually eliminating it first rather than last, as it may take the longest to wean you off of it. In fact, according to Dr. Neal Barnard, author of *Breaking the Food Seduction*, cheese is quite literally addictive and acts on the brain much like other drugs with a mild opiate-like effect. No wonder it's so hard to give up! The less you eat these addicting foods, the less you want them, so reducing your cheese consumption now is a great first step toward veganism, even if you're not already vegetarian.

If you've decided that you're motivated and disciplined enough to go "cold turkey" (or you just don't really care for milk and meat anyway), here's another piece of unconventional wisdom: Celebrate and indulge one last time. Eat your favorite nonvegan meal guilt-free. Just make sure there aren't any leftovers around if you're going vegan the next day!

Middle Path Transition

While quitting animal products cold turkey or doing a gradual elimination are both great transition methods, there is also a third way of going vegan that balances the two with a "middle path."

The "middle path" way to veganism recommends reducing your overall meat and dairy consumption while increasing consumption of plant-based foods. Think of this as a "prevegan" adjustment period. Take meat away from the center of your plate and put it on the side. Instead of a full steak, cook up a vegetarian stir-fry with lots of vegetables and a bit of beef over whole grains. Making a pepperoni pizza? Use half the amount of pepperoni you'd normally use, and pile on extra veggies. Don't give anything up completely, unless you're ready. Just reduce the quantity and portions of meat and dairy foods you eat while increasing your plant-based ingredients.

During this prevegan phase, eliminate or reduce whatever's easiest for you first, and you're not likely to miss it while you work on eliminating the other foods. For example, switch to soy or almond milk from dairy when cooking and baking and use vegan mayonnaise on sandwiches. You'll barely even notice both of these changes, even if you're not quite ready to make the leap from turkey sandwiches to Tofurky slices.

Before You Start

A week or so before you begin to transition to a vegan diet, start to prepare your kitchen. Gradually get rid of any nonvegan foods or condiments and start stocking up on vegan pantry items. (See Chapter 5: Ingredients for Healthy Vegan Cooking.)

Gather up a few reusable storage containers for leftovers and for transporting food and snacks with you. Even if you are at home during the day and don't need to worry about bringing lunch into the office, there will inevitably be some times when you'll need a meal or at least some snacks when you're out and about. Having something ready to go will make your life much easier.

New Twists on Familiar Favorites

If you have decided that a vegan diet makes sense for you and your lifestyle, you may want to start in slowly, learning what you need to eat and trying out the various vegan options in your market. Veggies and fruits are one thing, but what about all those different tofu and soy products? How do they fit in?

Plan a week's worth of menus, basing your main dishes on ones you love, but switching out, say, the beef meatballs for vegetarian ones. Or if you are a chili-head, why not create some really appealing meatless chilies, or for that meaty texture, add the taco-seasoned soy ground meat with plenty of beans and salsa for a satisfying entrée.

If cheese is your secret passion, try any of the shredded or sliced soy cheeses in your favorite recipes. These soy products not only taste and look like meats and dairy cheese; they also give nonvegans the sense that they can edge into their new diet without feeling deprived of their favorite foods. Even if you get derailed along the way and keep a few meats and seafood in your menus, you will still feel you've made the great vegan leap.

Vegan Meal Planning

Vegan meal planning centers around combining three basic ingredients: a grain or carbohydrate, a fruit or vegetable, and a protein. That doesn't mean you can't have a meal with more than one of each or some meals with only two, but it's a convenient way to think about creating well-balanced vegan meals. A simple vegetable stir-fry with tofu (protein) and brown rice (grain) would suit this plan perfectly, as would a bowl of whole grain cereal with soy milk (protein) and bananas.

Another way to plan healthy meals is to think of foods in fours, instead of threes. The Physicians Committee for Responsible Medicine (PCRM) divides healthy vegan foods into four equal categories: fruits, vegetables, legumes, and grains. The nutritionists at PCRM suggest that a day of vegan meals should be portioned relatively equally between these foods. If you can't easily identify which of these four groups a food belongs to, chances are it's been heavily processed and is a food you should be eating minimally.

Whichever way works best for you, whether in threes or fours, plan to get a wide variety within each food group. Broccoli is wonderfully nutritious, but you'll need to eat more vegetables than just broccoli in order to maintain a healthy and well-rounded diet. If you ate broccoli on Monday, try cauliflower on Tuesday and green beans on Wednesday. Similarly, don't rely on just one source of protein but eat a variety of nuts, beans and legumes, and lentils throughout the day and throughout the week.

Variety in Color

Need a convenient way to remember to vary your veggies? Remember this: eat the rainbow. Think of the colors of each fruit and vegetable—red strawberries, orange bell peppers, yellow squash, green romaine, blue blueberries, and purple eggplant—and try to incorporate each color from time to time. It may be oversimplifying what nutritionists surely spent years studying, but "eat the rainbow" is an easy way to remember that each color found in nature provides a different nutrient, and for a healthy variety of nutrients, a mishmash of colors is best.

Every day should include at least one serving of fresh, raw fruits or vegetables, such as raw veggies dipped in hummus or dressing, a green salad, or even just an apple. Obviously, the more fresh, raw, uncooked fruits and veggies you can include regularly, the better, and most days you'll easily get several servings rather than just one.

No matter what else you're eating, include several servings of green, leafy vegetables a week for optimum nutrition. There's just no substitute for fresh, raw, leafy greens, which are the most nutrient-dense foods on the planet. And finally, because it bears repeating, when planning your own vegan menus, don't forget that a healthy vegan diet requires a reliable source of vitamin B_{12}, preferably more than one.

Easy Go-To Meals

Like stir-fries and an easy pasta recipe, fried rice is a quick and easy vegan meal you can turn to again and again. The formula is always the same: rice, oil, and seasonings, but the variations are endless. Besides tofu, try adding tempeh, seitan, or store-bought mock meats to fried rice. Add kimchi for a Korean spice, or season with a mixture of cumin, curry, ginger, and turmeric for an Indian-inspired dish.

Snacks

Are you one of those people who gets the afternoon snack attacks and really needs something sweet, fast? Do you dare to go shopping when you are really, really hungry and end up buying way more than you can use or eat?

You can make wise choices to keep hunger at bay by stocking plenty of fresh fruits, protein and energy bars, and some homemade choices such as hummus and guacamole that you can enjoy with chips or pita slices. Other tasty options for the afternoon—or morning—doldrums are freshly popped popcorn sprinkled with herb seasonings; trail mix; a black, kidney, or pinto bean dip with taco chips; and bananas or slices of whole-grain bread slathered with peanut, cashew, or almond butter.

Vegan in a Nonvegan Family

Suppose that you are vegan but the rest of your household is not. You could micro-wave a veggie burger every night, but that's really not a solution. Your partner may want to try some vegan foods or even make some vegan meals for you. You need ideas for vegan foods that everyone will eat.

One approach that many vegans in this situation use is to make meatless dishes that you eat as entrées and that your family can use as side dishes if they want to.

Another idea is to make dishes you can eat as is and to which family can add meat or cheese. As you cook, just prepare a bit of meat separately and add it into only a portion of an otherwise vegan meal. For example, stir-fried vegetables can be supplemented with sautéed tofu or chicken. Cheese or cooked ground beef can be added to pasta sauce or chili.

If you make burritos or tacos, your portion can be filled with beans and veggies and your partner's with meat or cheese. Similarly, baked potatoes can be topped with a bean-based or meat-based sauce.

2

Understanding Vegan Nutrition

A plant-based diet offers many health benefits; however, it can be extremely challenging to sustain a nutritionally complete diet without eating animal products. But the good news is, it is possible, as long as you are intentional about what you eat. This chapter will help you understand the nutritional challenges of a vegan diet and give you a number of practical solutions.

Do your research and determine your individual goals. Which foods do you choose to eat? Perhaps there isn't a term that fits you exactly, and that is okay! What's important is that you feel comfortable and confident about your food choices. This chapter will help you create a well-balanced diet that suits you.

A Nutritionist Can Help

Because vegans eat no dairy products or eggs, their diets are often deficient in and even lack some basics, such as calcium from milk and vitamin B_{12}, a nutrient found exclusively in animal proteins.

A new vegan's best bet is to become familiar with the key nutrients and where to find them. It may also be worth consulting a registered dietitian or a nutritionist to get the pertinent nutritional information. If you make that choice, be sure to select someone who is well trained and who has had experience in counseling vegans and in planning a vegan menu.

With knowledge of body chemistry and an understanding of food science, that person can take a medical history and then question you about what you have been eating, why you are making the dietary change, and what your food likes and dislikes are. He or she will know your age and probably ask about your activity level; if you exercise regularly and are fairly active, your nutritional needs will be higher. Then you two can plan what your meals should include, so you can buy, cook, and eat the most wholesome foods.

Key Nutrients for Vegans

Whether you consult a dietitian or just map out your own vegan plan, you need to know some basics. Key nutrients include protein; vitamins D, B_{12}, and A; and minerals iron, calcium, and zinc. You will also need a source of omega-3 fatty acids, important for preventing heart disease.

Vegans may need to add dietary supplements to meet all their nutrient needs. Especially if you're a heavy smoker or coffee drinker, consider taking a supplement, as cigarettes and coffee inhibit absorption of several nutrients.

Also, consider fortified foods such as soy milk with added nutrients and fortified breakfast cereals to your daily menu plans. Many of today's foods are fortified with added vitamins and minerals. Fortifying milk with vitamin D is one example; adding folic acid to specific foods is another.

Vitamin D

Vitamin D is needed for your body to absorb calcium, so it is often linked to healthy bones.

Vitamin D is known as the sunshine vitamin because your body makes vitamin D when your skin is exposed to the sun.

It doesn't take much sun exposure to make all the vitamin D that you need. If you're fair-skinned and can be out in the summer sun, experts estimate that you need about 5 to 10 minutes a few times a week on your arms and face to meet your needs. This is a very rough estimate, however, and many factors can affect the production of vitamin D. If your skin is darker or if you live where there's a lot of air pollution or it's a cloudy day, you will need more sun exposure to make vitamin D. Winter sun in the northern part of the United States is not strong enough to promote vitamin D production.

Sunscreen and clothing block vitamin D production, so if you'd like to get vitamin D from the sun, wait a few minutes before putting on sunscreen or covering up. Remember though, that use of sunscreen is important to lower your risk for skin cancer.

Only a few foods contain vitamin D naturally—mushrooms are one example of a vegan food that provides some vitamin D. Some mushrooms that have recently become available are exposed to ultraviolet light, which increases their vitamin D content. The main dietary source of vitamin D for many Americans is the vitamin D added to cow's milk. Vegan sources of vitamin D are also fortified foods; vitamin D is added to some brands of plant milks, fruit juices, and breakfast cereals.

Vitamin D supplements are another option. Many calcium supplements also contain vitamin D. Before taking extra vitamin D (beyond what is in your prenatal), check with your healthcare provider or registered dietitian (RD) to make sure you're not overdoing this vitamin.

Calcium

Calcium is the key mineral needed for forming and maintaining strong bones and teeth, but it also helps it with other body functions. Almost every one of the food groups in a vegan's diet has foods that can markedly add to calcium intake. From nuts and seeds (almonds, sesame, tahini) to vegetables (okra, butternut squash), and fruit juices, foods from all of these groups as well as beans (black, great northern, navy, soy) and grains can provide calcium that is very well absorbed. Typically, about 30 percent of the calcium in dairy products is absorbed. That same 30 percent is absorbed from foods fortified with calcium. Green vegetables are the true prizewinners when it comes to calcium; more than half of the calcium in green vegetables like bok choy, broccoli, Chinese cabbage, collard greens, kale, mustard greens, and turnip greens is absorbed.

Many soy foods, such as tofu, soy milk, and TVP, are fortified with calcium. Before you pour a glass of fortified orange juice or soy milk, shake it up! The calcium in these drinks tends to settle at the bottom of the carton, so to get the best bone-boosting effect, shake before you drink.

To build strong bones, you need exercise as well as calcium, so vegan or not, diet is only half the equation.

Vegan Sources of Calcium

Vegans get calcium from different food groups rather than only one food group—dairy—as nonvegans do. Green leafy vegetables, fortified soy milk, and almonds are examples of some vegan calcium sources. The table below lists amounts of vegan foods that provide approximately 150 milligrams of calcium. By choosing at least six servings (6 × 150 = 900 mg) from this list and getting the rest of the calcium you need from other foods, you can meet the recommended daily allowance (RDA) of 1,000 milligrams of calcium. If you are taking a supplement that contains calcium, you will need fewer servings of calcium-rich foods.

Foods Supplying Approximately 150 mg of Calcium	
Food	**Serving Size**
Cooked collards or turnip greens	½ cup
Cooked kale or broccoli rabe	¾ cup
Cooked bok choy, okra, or mustard greens	1 cup
Cooked broccoli	1½ cups
Calcium-fortified juice (orange or vegetable) or milk (soy, almond, etc.)	4 ounces
Calcium-fortified vegan yogurt	3 ounces
Calcium-fortified vegan cheese	¾ ounce
Tofu	2 ounces
Tempeh	¾ cup
Almonds	6 tablespoons
Almond butter or tahini	2 tablespoons
Cooked dried beans	1½ cups (1 cup soybeans)
Dried figs	10
English muffin made with calcium propionate	1½
Blackstrap molasses	2 teaspoons
Calcium-fortified energy bar	½

Calcium Supplements

The two most common forms of calcium supplements are calcium carbonate and calcium citrate. Each kind has some advantages.

Calcium carbonate is usually less expensive, and fewer tablets may be needed. It is absorbed best when taken with food. The drawback of taking calcium supplements with foods is that the calcium interferes with iron absorption.

Calcium supplements made with calcium citrate can be taken between meals, so there's less chance that they'll interfere with iron absorption.

Calcium supplements may cause you to have more gas or to feel bloated or constipated. If that happens, try to take several smaller doses of calcium supplements throughout the day or try a different brand.

Very high intakes of calcium have been associated with kidney stones, not something anyone wants. It's unlikely you'll go over the safe upper limit for calcium of 2,500 milligrams a day from your diet, but if you're also taking calcium supplements, it can happen. Check the labels of all supplements for their calcium content.

Key Nutrients for Bone Health

Together, calcium and vitamin D are thought of as the most important nutrients for healthy bones, but other vitamins and minerals, along with protein, are also needed for bone health. When bones first develop, protein forms a sort of scaffolding that is filled in with the minerals calcium and phosphorus.

Calcium and phosphorus are what make bones hard and unlikely to break. Vitamin D plays an important role because it increases the amount of calcium that is absorbed. Your bones need a constant supply of calcium because they are always changing and rebuilding, even when you're no longer growing.

Other important nutrients for healthy bones include phosphorus, vitamin K, vitamin B_{12}, riboflavin, protein, and vitamin B_6. In other words, eating a well-balanced diet is one of the best things you can do to make sure that your bones get the nutrients they need.

Protein and Calcium

The relationship between protein, calcium, and bone health is a complex one. Older research suggested that people on very high-protein diets had a lot of calcium in their urine. In other words, they were losing calcium rather than storing it. This research led to the idea that people whose diets were lower in protein lost less calcium. Since their calcium losses were lower, the theory was that people on lower protein diets would not need as much calcium. Some vegans seized on this idea and guessed that vegans wouldn't need as much calcium as meat eaters do since the vegan diet is typically lower in protein.

More recent studies have found that both adequate protein and adequate calcium are needed to produce strong bones less likely to fracture. Vegans should try to meet the RDA for calcium and to have enough protein in their diets.

Iron

The body needs iron for red blood cells and carrying oxygen throughout the body. Iron deficiency leads to anemia, a condition characterized by fatigue, insomnia, and weakness, and one that commonly occurs in women and children.

When it comes to iron, most vegans and vegetarians actually get more than omnivores. Lentils, chickpeas, tahini, kidney beans, blackstrap molasses, and whole-wheat baked goods are good vegan sources of iron. Dark leafy greens such as spinach and kale are also excellent sources of not just iron but many other essential nutrients. These vegetables are one of the most nutrient-rich foods on the planet. Find ways to include kale, spinach, or other greens in your diet by snipping them into pasta sauces and casseroles, or include a few spinach leaves along with your other salad greens.

Iron Paired with Vitamin C

Nonheme iron, the only form of iron found in plants, is absorbed to a greater or lesser extent, depending on the other foods that are eaten along with plant sources of iron. Substances called phytates are major inhibitors of iron absorption. Phytates are found in a number of foods vegans commonly eat, including whole grains, dried beans, nuts, seeds, and vegetables. It may seem that almost every food that you think of as a good vegan iron source contains these substances that interfere with iron absorption.

The good news is that foods that provide vitamin C can pretty much counteract phytates' interfering actions. Something as simple as drinking a small glass of orange juice with a meal can increase the amount of iron absorbed as much as 400 percent, even if phytates are present.

It's not just orange juice that can help increase iron absorption. All citrus fruits and juices provide vitamin C. So do tomatoes and tomato products (tomato sauce, tomato juice, and tomato soup), broccoli, cauliflower, cabbage, cantaloupe, kiwi, pineapple, kale, sweet potatoes—most fruits and many vegetables can add vitamin C.

Foods That Inhibit Iron Absorption

Coffee (both regular and decaffeinated), tea (including some herbal teas), and cocoa contain substances that interfere with iron absorption. If you use these beverages, wait to have them until several hours have gone by after a meal with a lot of iron in it to keep substances in the beverages from blocking your body's uptake of that iron.

Calcium supplements can also interfere with iron absorption. If you're taking calcium pills, take them between meals.

Zinc

Have you heard about taking a zinc supplement if you begin to feel sick? That's because the mineral zinc helps bolster the immune system. But as the Office of Dietary Supplements at the National Institutes of Health in Bethesda, Maryland, points out, zinc also helps heal wounds and helps sustain the senses of smell and taste. Vegans can source zinc from beans, nuts, and whole grains.

The following vegan foods are especially good zinc sources:

- Zinc-fortified breakfast cereals (up to 15 milligrams of zinc in 1 ounce of cereal)
- Wheat germ (2.7 milligrams in 2 tablespoons)
- Zinc-fortified veggie "meats" (up to 1.8 milligrams in 1 ounce)
- Zinc-fortified energy bars (up to 5.2 milligrams in a bar)
- Adzuki beans (4 milligrams in 1 cup)
- Tahini (1.4 milligrams in 2 tablespoons)
- Chickpeas (2.4 milligrams in 1 cup)
- Black-eyed peas (2.2 milligrams in 1 cup)
- Lentils (2.6 milligrams in 1 cup)
- Peanuts, peanut butter (close to 2 milligrams in 2 tablespoons)

Zinc Absorption

While zinc absorption is lower from beans and grains than it is from meats, there are definitely techniques that you can use to raise the amount of zinc you absorb from a vegan diet. Zinc is better absorbed from yeast-raised breads than from quick breads or muffins that are leavened with baking powder or baking soda. That doesn't mean that you can't eat quick breads or muffins; just be aware that yeast-raised breads provide more zinc. Zinc absorption is higher from fermented foods like sauerkraut, soy sauce, and tempeh. If you are into sprouting, you're in luck. Sprouting grains and beans reduces their phytate content and makes it easier to absorb the zinc in these foods.

Omega-3 Fatty Acids

Fish oils and fish such as salmon are often touted as a source of healthy omega-3 fatty acids, but vegans can obtain these from flaxseeds and flaxseed oil, as well as walnuts or hemp seeds.

Flaxseeds are small, dark brown seeds with a slightly nutty taste. You can find them in breakfast cereals, breads, and even snack crackers and tortilla chips. Whole flaxseeds add a nice crunch, but that's about all; the fact is that most of them pass through your body undigested because of their hull. In order to release the omega-3 fatty acids from flaxseeds, the seeds need to be ground into flaxseed meal, a powder that can be used in baking or added to smoothies. You can grind your own using a spice or coffee grinder or purchase it already ground. Flaxseed meal should be stored in the refrigerator or freezer.

Hemp seeds and hemp seed oil come from the hemp plant. You may have noticed hemp seeds, hemp milk, hemp flour, hemp oil, and hemp butter as well as products with added hemp at the grocery store. Shelled hemp seeds can be sprinkled onto foods or used in baking. Hemp seed butter can be used in place of peanut butter, and hemp flour is a gluten-free product.

Best Uses for Flaxseed Oil

Flaxseed oil has a sweet and nutty flavor. Never use it as a cooking oil, however, as the heat destroys the healthy fats and creates unhealthy free radicals. Instead, add a teaspoonful of flax oil to your favorite salad dressing or drizzle it over already cooked dishes for your daily quota of omega-3s. Look for a brand that is cold-pressed and store chilled to keep it fresh. Flaxseed oil is added to many foods. If you'd like to get more omega-3 fats, look for peanut butter or vegan margarine with added flaxseed oil. Of course, you can make your own flaxseed oil–enhanced peanut butter by mixing a spoonful of flaxseed oil with a couple of spoonfuls of peanut butter.

Vitamin B_{12}

Your body may need only small amounts of vitamin B_{12}, but it is essential for the proper growth of red blood cells and for the health of some nerve tissues. Signs of a B_{12} deficiency include numbness and tingling in hands and legs, weakness, disorientation, and depression, among others.

Vitamin B_{12} cannot reliably be obtained from vegan foods. Deficiencies of this important nutrient are admittedly rare, and if you're eating vegan meals only occasionally, you don't need to worry. Vegetarians will absorb B_{12} from food sources, but long-term vegans, and pregnant and breastfeeding women, in particular, need a reliable source. Take a supplement and eat fortified foods, such as nutritional yeast. One brand, Red Star's Vegetarian Support Formula nutritional yeast, is a reliable source of vitamin B_{12}.

Because the body needs very little B_{12}, and it can be stored for years, some people claim a supplement is not needed or suggest that omnivores are more likely to be deficient in a variety of nutrients, and thus the B_{12} issue for vegans is grossly overblown. Although this last argument may be true, the bottom line, according to most experts, is to take a supplement. Better safe than sorry.

If you're taking vitamin B_{12} in pill form, it should be crushed or chewed before swallowing. This improves the odds that the B_{12} in the pill will be well absorbed. Crushed B_{12} pills can be mixed with applesauce, pudding, or other foods to minimize the taste. Powdered B_{12} in vegan capsules does not need to be chewed.

Vegan Foods Commonly Fortified with Vitamin B$_{12}$

While Vitamin B$_{12}$ cannot reliably be obtained from vegan foods, fortunately for vegans many food manufacturers add vitamin B$_{12}$ to their products—check labels to see if vitamin B$_{12}$ is added to foods you use. Some vegan products that commonly (or at least sometimes) have vitamin B$_{12}$ added are:

- Plant milks
- Energy bars and protein bars
- Marmite yeast extract
- Tofu
- Vegetarian Support Formula nutritional yeast
- Veggie "meats"
- Breakfast cereals

Companies have been known to change their product formulation, especially with regard to vitamin fortification. Check the labels of foods you rely on for vitamin B$_{12}$ frequently, so you're not lulled into thinking a product has vitamin B$_{12}$ when it no longer does.

Myths about Vitamin B$_{12}$ Sources

Foods reported to contain vitamin B$_{12}$ include fermented foods (tempeh, sauerkraut, miso), sea vegetables, shiitake mushrooms, spirulina (algae), and soybeans. None of these foods—in fact, no plant foods—contain enough B$_{12}$ to prevent a deficiency. In fact, some of these foods contain a vitamin B$_{12}$ analogue (something that looks like vitamin B$_{12}$ but isn't) that can interfere with B$_{12}$ absorption from other foods.

Vitamin Excess

Vitamin and mineral supplements may seem like harmless pills. They are available without a prescription and may be something you take without much thought. In reality, taking too much of some vitamins and minerals can cause health problems. The simplest way to avoid a problem is to only take the vitamins and minerals that have been approved by your doctor.

Dietary supplements are meant to supplement your diet; they do not take the place of eating a healthy, varied vegan diet.

Nutrient-Dense Foods

Eating a variety of foods is always good advice. That way, if one food that you eat is high in vitamin X but low in mineral Y, you're likely to choose another food that will be low in vitamin X but high in mineral Y. Eating a variety of foods lets you relax and not have to worry about keeping track of every nutrient.

Certain foods in each food group are especially good sources of a variety of nutrients. For example, in the grains group, whole grains supply more fiber and more of some vitamins and minerals than their refined counterparts.

In the vegetables group, dark-green vegetables and deep-orange vegetables are your best choice. That doesn't mean iceberg lettuce and mushrooms are off-limits, just that these less nutrient-rich foods should be balanced with some carrots and kale.

Fresh fruits provide more fiber than more processed fruits or juices. If you choose to use canned fruits, select fruits packed in fruit juice rather than in heavy syrup. Dried beans, tofu, tempeh, soy milk, nuts, and nut butters are excellent choices from the protein-rich foods group. More processed foods like veggie "meats" are often higher in sodium, lower in fiber, and more expensive.

Foods to Limit

Everything in moderation is a standard piece of nutrition advice. While moderation is a reasonable approach to eating, be sure that you know what "moderation" means. Moderation means that after you have eaten the appropriate amounts of nutrient-rich foods, it's all right to have a small (emphasis on small) amount of what are often called junk foods.

Junk foods are foods that you would be just fine, nutritionally speaking, if you never ate them again. The sole nutritional value of these foods is that they provide calories; they're not great sources of protein, vitamins, minerals, or other things you need.

Examples of junk foods are soft drinks, candy, cookies, cake, chips, and greasy snack foods. Remember, just because a food is vegan doesn't mean it's healthy. What's wrong with these foods?

Think of your eating plan like your household budget—you have to make choices to stay on your budget. You need a certain amount of calories to support a healthy weight; you don't want to "spend" those calories on nonnutritious foods. Rather, you want to get the best nutrition possible within your allotted calories. If you overdo junk foods, they can displace healthier foods in your diet—not good for you.

Processed Foods

To ensure you're receiving the maximum nutrition available from the foods you eat, avoid processed foods and select, instead, the whole foods that are complete as nature intended them. Processed grains, sugars, and flours are often stripped of their natural nutrients. Even when vitamins and minerals are added back in later—a process called "enriching," which means the nutrients lost during refining are added back in to enrich the product—the total effect is never the same.

White rice, for example, may cook faster and have a more adaptable taste, but by stripping away the outer bran layer, the rice grains lose much of their beneficial fiber and minerals. As proof, 1 cup of brown rice contains 3.5 grams of fiber. One cup of white rice contains less than 1 gram. Even enriching white rice doesn't make up the difference in the loss of fiber and minerals.

Enriching means putting back into a refined food the nutrients lost during processing; fortifying means perhaps putting back lost nutrients but also adding others that may not occur naturally in a particular food.

Processing or refining plant foods can also destroy the complex plant chemicals known as phytonutrients, or phytochemicals. Many of these naturally occurring chemicals have health-supporting benefits and have been consumed for centuries for their antioxidant, anti-inflammatory, and anticarcinogenic properties. Considering that salicin, extracted from the white willow tree, has long been recognized as a painkiller and the basis for today's aspirin, it's easy to understand why unprocessed fruits and vegetables can be your body's best friends.

Organic Foods

In 2002, the USDA label was implemented and replaced private organic labeling programs. A concern arose about the level of standards in the new label after synthetic additive traces were found in products such as baby food. The demand for organic food products has tremendously increased, and the industry has expanded to a $20 billion per year business. The label is no longer a guarantee that consumers can trust, however. In general, limiting processed foods and purchasing from local farmers is the safest way to consume most of your organic food.

Confusion about whether to buy organic or not in the produce section may be a factor in the lack of organic fruit and vegetable consumption in the United States. According to the USDA Economic Research Service, vegetable consumption is not meeting the recommendations in the *Dietary Guidelines for Americans 2015–2020*. The higher cost of organic foods may also overwhelm some consumers. A need existed for a simple tool to help consumers feel confident in their purchases, so the Environmental Working Group has provided the public with their Shopper's Guide to Pesticides, updated in 2018. You can view the guide at www.foodnews.org. This is a great resource for consumers who would like to improve their health.

The fruits and vegetables found lowest in pesticides, according to the Clean Fifteen from the Environmental Working Group are:

- Avocados
- Sweet corn
- Pineapples
- Cabbages
- Onions
- Sweet peas, frozen
- Papayas
- Asparagus
- Mangos
- Eggplants
- Honeydew melons
- Kiwis
- Cantaloupes
- Cauliflower
- Broccoli

3

Plant Protein Is Your Friend

A strict vegan diet excludes all animal products. You may wonder where vegans get their protein with no meat or even dairy in their diet. There are plenty of plant-based protein sources perfect for the vegan diet, and this chapter will help you understand them.

Protein, whether it comes from an animal or a plant, is one of the macronutrients and most important sources of calories to be consumed at each meal, including snacks. Its power to slow digestion and regulate blood sugars, hunger, and energy levels can improve your productivity and performance—and you won't need to take so many coffee breaks. This is especially true during that afternoon drop when many of us reach for a quick fix of processed foods or "empty calories."

Protein in a Healthy Diet

Protein builds and maintains muscles, organs, connective tissues, skin, bones, teeth, blood, and your DNA (deoxyribonucleic acid). It helps the body heal when it is sick, wounded, or depleted. Without protein, even mild exercise would weaken you to the point of exhaustion.

Protein contributes to the formation of enzymes. Almost all reactions that occur in the body, such as digestion, require enzymes. Enzymes are catalysts to these reactions, increasing the rate at which they occur.

There is protein in your blood, called antibodies. They serve as your body's immune responders. They bind with and fight foreign invaders, such as bacteria or toxins. Protein is found in hormones, your body's chemical messengers. Hormones help regulate the body's activities, maintaining balance, or homeostasis.

Protein Defined

Protein is composed of twenty amino acids. These acids link together in chains to form the variety of proteins your body needs. The length and shape of the chain determine the protein's structure. Of the twenty amino acids, eleven of them are made by your body. These eleven acids are called nonessential because you do not need to consume them. The remaining nine amino acids are called essential, and it is important that you eat these every day. Getting all nine essential amino acids is not hard, especially if you eat meat. Animal foods (which include meat, eggs, and dairy products) contain the largest concentration of protein. Animal protein is considered complete because it contains all nine essential amino acids.

Plant foods also contain proteins. Quinoa, soy, and hemp seeds are vegan powerhouses for protein, as they contain the highest amount of all nine essential amino acids. Hemp seeds are also high in omega-3 and omega-6 essential fatty acids.

But few plants contain complete protein. This is one of the challenges of veganism because to stay healthy you must consume enough foods with the right mixture of amino acids. It sounds complicated, but grains, nuts, and legumes contain the proteins that are not found in other plants, so adding a variety of these to your diet does the trick.

Complementary Proteins

Plant foods eaten in combination to create complete protein are called complementary proteins. When these foods are eaten over the course of a day, protein intake is complete. Protein derived from complementary plant proteins is considered a healthy alternative and, by many people, a superior one. Eating such combinations of plant foods not only completes the protein but also provides other nutrients vital to good health as well, most notably fiber, vitamins, and minerals. And most plants do all that without saturated fat.

Eating complementary protein means consuming both beans and grains every day. The beans can be pinto, kidney, black, lentils, garbanzo, split peas, or peanuts. Grains should be whole, including brown rice, whole-wheat pasta, bread, crackers, or tortillas. Sesame seeds also complement the protein of beans.

Amino Acids in Plant-Based Protein

In 1971, Frances Moore Lappé wrote a book that revolutionized the relationship thousands of Americans had with their plates, effectively launching vegetarianism into the public consciousness. *Diet for a Small Planet* continues to be a widely read and cited book today. Much to the chagrin of generations of vegetarians, however, it was the beginning of a myth still oft retold. This is the myth of "protein combining," or the idea that plant sources provide "incomplete" proteins whereas meats provide "complete" proteins.

Lappé theorized that in order to digest all nine of the essential amino acids the human body needs to build protein, vegetarians needed to combine foods so as to consume each essential amino acid in one sitting. Whole grains needed to be consumed at the same time as nuts, for example. The truth is, by eating a variety of foods, you'll have nothing to worry about. Although you do need a full range of amino acids, and some plant-based foods contain more or less of the essentials, Lappé's error was assuming these nine essentials must be consumed at the same meal. Nutritionists, including the Academy of Nutrition and Dietetics and the USDA, have since refuted this claim, and even Lappé herself revised her stance in later editions of the book. Your body will store and combine proteins on its own.

If, however, you tend to go weeks eating nothing but bananas and soda, you'll quickly find yourself deficient in more than just protein. But eat a relatively healthy diet and you'll be just fine. According to the Academy of Nutrition and Dietetics, "Plant sources of protein alone can provide adequate amounts of the essential and nonessential amino acids, assuming that dietary protein sources from plants are reasonably varied."

Protein Needs

The word *protein* comes from the Greek word *prōteios*, meaning "primary." Perhaps this word was chosen because of protein's primary role in body function. Proteins are responsible for everything from the structure of your muscles and bones to the proper function of your immune system to food digestion. Many hormones are made from protein. Adequate protein is needed for healthy skin, hair, and nails.

The average person needs around 0.4 grams of protein for every pound of body weight. The math isn't hard to do. Take your weight in pounds and multiply by 0.4 to calculate how much protein you need each day. For instance, a person who weighs 120 pounds would multiply 120 by 0.4 (calculators allowed, this is not a test) and get 48 grams of protein. Pregnant women need to increase their daily protein intake by about 25 grams each day starting in the fourth month of pregnancy.

Some vegan nutrition experts recommend that vegans get slightly more protein than nonvegans. Their rationale is that vegan protein sources like beans and whole grains are harder to digest. They suggest about 10 percent more protein for vegans. This amount is pretty small and is nothing to be concerned about. If you want to calculate, multiply your protein recommendation by 1.1.

The Disadvantages of Meat

Meat is generally considered a high-fat protein choice. Usually fat means flavor. In today's world people appreciate, and even expect, a high level of flavor in their meat, despite full knowledge that saturated fat contributes to coronary artery disease and elevated cholesterol levels.

Lean cuts are available, but even if you cannot see the fat marbled throughout a particular cut, the saturated fat is still present within the muscle cells. When meat is heated, the fat melts and penetrates the muscle. So even if you do not eat the visible fat on a steak, you are consuming saturated fat.

This appetite for fatty beef has drastically changed the landscape of modern agriculture. Today cattle are bred and raised to provide the most meat with the least cost. According to the USDA, the average American consumes 67 pounds of beef every year.

A wild cow would naturally consume fiber-rich plants that are unsuitable for human consumption. Today, cows compete with humans for food, consuming grain grown on valuable fertile soil. In the United States, half of the water and 80 percent of the grain harvested goes to feed livestock.

Vegan Protein Sources

Some vegan foods that are especially high in protein are soybeans, tempeh, and lentils. These foods have 20 or more grams of protein in a serving—1 cup of beans or 4 ounces of tempeh. Other foods that provide generous amounts of protein (10–20 grams per serving) include tofu, veggie burgers, and cooked dried beans. Soy milk, peanut butter, soy yogurt, and quinoa are all good sources of protein as well. Vegetables, whole grains, pasta, almond butter, and nuts and seeds are other good foods to add to your protein intake.

Vegan and Nonvegan Protein Comparison Chart

These two charts list the protein content for vegan and nonvegan foods. As you can see, many plant-based foods contain just as much protein as animal-based foods.

Sources of Vegan Protein		
Food	**Serving Size**	**Protein (grams)**
Edamame	1 cup	22.2
MorningStar Farms burger crumbles	1 cup	21.2
Vital wheat gluten	1 ounce	21.0
Tempeh	4 ounces (½ block)	20.4
Canned white beans	1 cup	19.0
Cooked lentils	1 cup	17.9
Chickpeas	1 cup	14.5
Tofu	½ (12-ounce) block	13.3
Pumpkin seeds	1 ounce	9.4
Quinoa, cooked	1 cup	8.1
Soy milk	1 cup	8.0
Peanut butter	2 tablespoons	8.0
Frozen spinach	1 cup	7.6
Whole-wheat pasta, cooked	1 cup	7.5
Wild rice, cooked	1 cup	6.4

Extracted from the USDA National Nutrient Database and https://ndb.nal.usda.gov/ndb/. Recommended dietary allowance is 56 grams for men, 46 grams for women.

Nonvegan Sources of Protein		
Food	Serving Size	Protein (grams)
Low-fat cottage cheese	1 cup	31.0
Chicken	½ breast	22.2
Cooked ground beef	3 ounces	21.7
Canned tuna fish	3 ounces	21.7
Fast-food hamburger	1 sandwich	13.9
Canned chicken soup	1 cup	12.3
Low-fat yogurt	8 ounces	9.9
2% milk	1 cup	8.1
Mozzarella cheese	1 ounce	7.4
Cooked bacon	3 slices	7.0
Egg	1 medium	5.5

Protein from Beans

The general term *bean* encompasses several plants and usually refers to the legume, a large plant seed found within long pods from the plant family Fabaceae. Soybeans, peas, lentils, and kidney beans are examples of legumes. When the seeds are dried, they are referred to as pulses. Many beans are only sold in dry form, although some, such as the pea, come both dried and fresh. As a valuable source of protein, few foods can equal what legumes have to offer. According to the Linus Pauling Institute at Oregon State University, legumes not only provide protein; they also supply micronutrients, minerals, fiber, and good carbs. Legumes contain little fat and no cholesterol, making them important elements for heart health and weight management.

Beans contain more than twice the amount of protein as grain. You can buy beans in dried or canned form. Dried beans take longer to cook and must first undergo a long soaking process to tenderize them. Canned beans are readily available, which makes it easy to add beans to your everyday diet. Most supermarkets stock such common beans as adzuki, black, broad bean, cannellini, chickpeas, fava, garbanzo, kidney, lentil, lima, mung, navy, pea, pinto, runner, soy, and white.

Protein from Nuts

Botanically, a nut is a fruit with one seed. The wall of the seed becomes very hard, and the meat of the seed stays very loose within. Walnuts, pecans, hazelnuts, and chestnuts fall into this category. However, in the world of cuisine there are other nuts that do not fit the definition. Peanuts are legumes, the pine nut is a seed from a pine tree, a macadamia nut is a kernel, and the Brazil nut is found inside a fruit capsule.

Nuts—from Brazil nuts, cashews, and hazelnuts to pecans—are rich in phytochemicals; they actually protect against heart disease, diabetes, and certain cancers. Besides, nuts are rich in both vitamins and minerals. Nuts contain the heart-healthy mono- and polyunsaturated fats, omega-3 fats, and arginine, all of which play a key role in benefiting the heart and keeping it healthy. But because nuts are calorie rich, people should cut way back on other fatty foods, keeping their nut intake to about 1 ounce a day, according to the FDA.

Nuts have a high oil content and can easily become rancid if stored improperly. Heat and light increase rancidity, so refrigeration is best for long-term storage. Flavor is greatly altered, and generally improved, by heat. Toasting nuts in an oven yields the best results. Spread them out on a baking sheet and roast at 350°F for 10–15 minutes, until they become fragrant. Nuts and seeds are extremely versatile and lend both texture and flavor to stews, sandwiches, desserts, soups, and stews, plus many other recipes.

Protein from Wild Rice

Wild rice is not actually rice but rather is the seed of a grass native to the Great Lakes region in the United States. With almost 7 grams of protein per cup when cooked, wild rice can be an excellent source of protein. Add ¼ cup wild rice per 1 cup of white rice to any recipe that calls for regular white rice for an extra protein boost.

Typically, the rice requires thorough rinsing and lengthy cooking to tenderize the grains. But some markets now sell precooked wild rice in vacuum-sealed foil packets that require only a few moments of reheating to ready it for the table.

Protein in Every Meal

There are some easy ways to incorporate good sources of protein into your daily meal plan. These are all highly nutritious foods, so by adding them you're adding not just protein but a host of vitamins and minerals as well.

At Breakfast

- Spread some peanut butter or other nut butter on your toast or bagel; peanut butter can even top oatmeal—add a spoonful of jelly for PB and J oatmeal.
- Blend soft or silken tofu with soy milk and fruit (fresh, frozen, or canned) for a quick smoothie.
- Use soy milk in place of water to prepare hot cereals.
- Mix things up with a bowl of quinoa instead of oatmeal.
- Replace water or other liquids in your favorite muffin and pancake recipes with soy milk.
- On more leisurely mornings try a tofu scramble or quiche for breakfast.

At Lunch

- Toss some chickpeas or black beans with your salad.
- Use a flavored hummus in place of mayo as a savory sandwich spread.
- Prepare a vegan cream soup with soy milk.
- Add extra crunch to a peanut butter sandwich by sprinkling on coarsely chopped peanuts or other nuts.
- Pack protein-rich leftovers to reheat at lunchtime.

At Dinner

- Purée white beans or soft tofu with your favorite tomato sauce and serve over whole-grain pasta.
- Top baked potatoes with a spoonful of plain soy yogurt and some chopped chives.
- A peanut sauce (homemade or purchased) can top rice, pasta, or vegetables.
- Add chickpeas or vegan pepperoni to take out or homemade veggie no-cheese pizza.

- Experiment with quinoa in dishes that use rice or other grains.
- Toss vegan stir-fry strips or homemade seitan with stir-fried vegetables.

For Snacks

- Make a batch of trail mix using a variety of nuts and dried fruits. Add soy nuts for a protein boost.
- Spread apple or pear slices with nut butters.
- Dip baby carrots and jicama strips into hummus or refried beans.
- Try different brands of vegan energy bars until you find one or more that suit you.
- Eat breakfast for a snack by having a bowl of cold cereal with soy milk.

Protein Supplements

Protein supplements come in different forms, most commonly powders that are mixed with water or other liquids. Vegan protein supplements do exist and are usually based on soy, rice, or hemp protein. If you are eating a varied vegan diet that includes good sources of protein, it's unlikely that any protein supplement is needed. Of course, if you have a number of food restrictions because of allergies or intolerances or have especially high protein needs because of a medical condition, your RD may suggest using protein supplements. For most vegans, however, they are an unnecessary expense.

4

Benefits, Risks, and Concerns of the Vegan Diet

Personal health is a strong motivator to eat a vegan diet. Medical research and the Academy of Nutrition and Dietetics affirm that a plant-based diet prevents many ailments, helps reverse some, and eases the symptoms of others.

From significantly reduced rates of hypertension, arterial hardening, stroke, type 2 diabetes, obesity, heart disease, and several types of cancer (prostate and breast cancer being the best documented), a plant-based diet helps prevent the vast majority of life-threatening diseases that plague modernity.

This chapter will detail the health benefits of the vegan diet and also address risks and common concerns associated with the diet.

Top Ten Health Benefits of a Vegan Diet

1. Vegans are less likely to become obese.
2. Vegans are less likely to develop coronary heart disease.
3. Vegans are less likely to develop high blood pressure.
4. Vegans are less likely to develop diabetes.
5. Vegans are less likely to suffer from certain cancers.
6. Vegans may develop less osteoporosis.
7. Vegans may suffer less from constipation.
8. Vegans may develop fewer gallstones.
9. Vegans are more likely to feel better and stay slimmer.
10. Vegans are likely to live longer.

Avoid Hormones in Foods

One benefit of the vegan diet is less exposure to hormones in foods. Hormone use is a major concern in much of the world, though the American public and lawmakers are less aware of the dangers. In the US, dairy cows are fed the drug "recombinant bovine growth hormone" (rBGH), which increases milk production up to 20 percent. Because this powerful hormone ends up in consumers' stomachs, Japan, Australia, Canada, and the European Union have banned the use of rBGH, and the European Union bans the import of American beef because of it. Medical studies implicate these hormones in the connection between diet and cancer, particularly breast, prostate, and testicular cancers.

High-Fiber Diet

Most Americans eat far less fiber each day than they should, but the vegan diet is full of fiber-rich foods. A type of carbohydrate, fiber is found in all plant foods, including whole grains and legumes, and is an indigestible carbohydrate. It occurs in two forms: insoluble fiber, which helps prevent constipation; and soluble fiber, which helps lower blood cholesterol levels. Fiber plays several important roles in your health by adding the roughage, or bulk, that keeps your digestive tract working smoothly. Because your body cannot absorb or digest it, fiber also slows down the digestive process so that glucose gets absorbed more slowly, and that helps keep blood sugar levels stable and reduces the risks of obesity and certain cancers.

Women should eat about 20 grams of fiber each day; men, 30-plus grams. All plants contain fiber, but some, such as beans, potatoes, and apples, are richer sources than others. When possible, eat your fruits and vegetables unpeeled or whole to receive the maximum fiber content.

Lower Cholesterol Levels

A study in the UK found that both lifelong vegetarians and vegans had lower levels of total and LDL cholesterol in their blood. LDL cholesterol is often referred to as "bad" cholesterol because it is associated with a higher risk of heart disease. When compared to vegetarians who ate eggs and dairy products, vegans had the lowest levels of total and LDL cholesterol. Based on their blood cholesterol levels, the incidence of heart disease might be 24 percent lower in lifelong vegetarians and 57 percent lower in lifelong vegans compared to meat eaters.

Improved Blood Pressure

High blood pressure increases the risk of developing heart disease and of having a stroke. Vegans tend to have lower blood pressure than meat eaters and a lower risk of developing hypertension (high blood pressure). Several studies have used vegan or near-vegan diets to treat people with heart disease. Results have been very positive in terms of modifying risk factors like obesity and LDL cholesterol levels.

As an added bonus for men (and for women too, really), it's possible that vegans really do make better lovers. High blood pressure, high cholesterol, and particularly the decreased blood flow associated with blocked arteries are common causes leading to erectile dysfunction, and vegans certainly have fewer instances of these symptoms.

Lower Body Weight and Reduced Risk of Type 2 Diabetes

One significant health advantage for vegans is that they tend to have lower body weights than either other vegetarians or meat eaters. Since being overweight increases the risk of developing many chronic diseases including heart disease, type 2 diabetes, high blood pressure, and even breast cancer, the lower average weight seen in vegans is a definite plus.

Vegans also have lower rates of type 2 diabetes. Type 2 diabetes is the most common form of diabetes. Risk factors for type 2 diabetes include a poor diet, excess weight, and little exercise. Low-fat vegan diets have been successfully used to treat type 2 diabetes.

Benefits Come from Balance

You do need to eat a balanced diet in order to reap these benefits. After all, French fries and potato chips are animal-free, but that doesn't make them healthy. So, what exactly constitutes a balanced vegan diet? According to Katherine Tallmadge, author of *Diet Simple*, past spokesperson for the Academy of Nutrition and Dietetics, immediate past president of the DC Metro Area Dietetic Association, and a practicing nutritionist, the daily diet program presented here, based on the ADA guidelines, should guide vegans to eat right.

Milk Alternatives Group:
Six to Eight Servings Daily

- ½ cup fortified soy milk
- ¼ cup calcium-set tofu
- 1 cup cooked dry beans, such as soy, cannellini, pinto, navy, great northern, kidney, and black beans
- ¼ cup shelled almonds
- 3 tablespoons sesame tahini or almond butter
- 1 cup cooked or 2 cups raw bok choy, Chinese cabbage, broccoli, collards, kale, or okra
- 1 tablespoon blackstrap molasses
- 5 figs

Dry Beans, Nuts, Seeds, Eggs, and Meat Substitutes Group:
Two to Three Servings Daily

- 1 cup cooked dry beans, lentils, or peas
- 2 cups soy milk
- ½ cup tofu or tempeh
- 2 ounces vegetarian "meats" or soy cheese
- ¼ cup nuts or seeds
- 3 tablespoons nut or seed butters

Fruit Group: Two to Four Servings Daily

- ¾ cup juice
- ¼ cup dried fruit
- ½ cup chopped raw fruit
- ½ cup canned fruit
- 1 medium-sized piece of fruit such as banana, apple, or orange

Vegetable Group: Three to Five Servings Daily

- ½ cup cooked or chopped raw vegetables
- 1 cup raw, leafy vegetables
- ¾ cup vegetable juice

Bread, Cereal, Rice, and Pasta Group:
Six to Eleven Servings Daily

- 1 slice (1 ounce) bread
- ½ small bagel, bun, or English muffin (about 1 ounce)
- 1 ounce ready-to-eat cereal
- 2 tablespoons wheat germ
- ½ cup cooked (1 ounce dry) grains, cereal, rice, or pasta

Fats, Oils, and Sweets: Use Sparingly

- Candy, solid margarine (high in trans fats)

Global Good

The health benefits of reduced animal consumption aren't just personal; they're global as well. The powerful cocktail of hormones and antibiotics pumped into cows and chickens by today's food industry ends up right back in local water supplies and affects everyone, even vegans. All these antibiotics, combined with the cramped conditions on modern farms, lead to dangerous new drug-resistant pathogens and bacterial strains. Swine flu, bird flu, SARS, and mad cow disease are all traced back to intense animal agriculture practices. Because of our rapidly shrinking planet, the "butterfly effect" is a very real phenomenon: a pig in Mexico sneezed, and a child in Bangkok died.

Pathogens in Raw Foods

Some vegans and vegetarians follow a raw-foods diet, but they should take special care with the fruits and vegetables they eat. According to the CDC, raw animal foods—including eggs and raw milk—may contain pathogens. But CDC scientists point out that any raw food exposed to a contaminated food source can contain pathogens.

Likewise, pathogens can readily contaminate raw fruits and vegetables, particularly if these were processed in unsanitary conditions, were fertilized with contaminated manure, or were washed for packing in unclean water. Even unpasteurized fruit juices may be unsafe if made from contaminated fresh fruits. Washing whole fresh produce at home may diminish but not totally eliminate any pathogens.

Proper Produce Washing

You are just back from the market with a bagful of goodies. The apples look clean, and you see only a few grains of dirt on the lettuce. Into the fridge right away? No. All produce needs a rinse-off before use; you can't be sure how it's grown or who has handled it before you bring it home. Besides, most produce—especially leafy greens such as lettuce and spinach—benefits from a little extra moisture before refrigeration. Just don't use soap and hot water!

While root vegetables need a scrubbing with a brush to clean off dirt, other vegetables and fruits can be swirled through a basin or tub of cold water, dried off with paper towels, and wrapped carefully in more paper towels and plastic—and, of course, refrigerated. Even though veggies labeled as prewashed may be safe enough to eat without extra rinsing, why take a chance? Give them a quick rinsing and drying off. Rinsing and wrapping also applies to fresh herbs, even to the herbs picked from your own garden.

Dietary Supplements

Since vegans may feel their diet lacks certain nutrients, they may reach for the vitamin or mineral pill to fill in the gaps. According to the FDA, supplements should not be used to replace a balanced diet. Consumers should also be aware that those with particular health problems and who are taking supplements may face some unintended results: the supplements may interact with prescription or over-the-counter drugs, or for the presurgical patient a supplement may cause dangerous interactions during surgery. For these reasons, it's important to seek medical or healthcare advice before taking any supplements. For further information, check out the Office of Dietary Supplements website at https://ods.od.nih.gov.

Soy and Your Health

Somewhere along the way, people realized that the soybean—besides its protein content—had other nutritional benefits as well: it contains few saturated fats; has no cholesterol; and provides isoflavones, minerals, and fiber. Some believe that all these characteristics make soy an effective disease fighter, working hard to combat certain cancers, strokes, and heart disease. Some point out that, as a rule, Asians suffer from fewer of these diseases than Westerners, with their rich meaty diets, and they believe that soy consumption is one reason for that. Other studies suggest that soy's properties may also combat osteoporosis, type 2 diabetes, and even obesity.

But, as it turns out, while some people describe soy as a "miracle" food, some skeptics challenge the prevalent notion that soy should be a staple in everyone's diet, replacing meat partially or totally. If you scroll through the web, you'll find plenty of conflicting arguments about the pros and cons of soy that will leave you completely mystified.

The Health Benefits of Soy

You've likely heard mixed messages about the health benefits of soy. Previous studies led to a 1999 ruling in which the FDA authorized food manufacturers to label their soy-based food—foods made with the whole soybean without any added fats and that contain at least 6.25 grams of soy protein per serving—as beneficial for keeping hearts healthy.

In a 2000 *FDA Consumer* magazine article titled "Soy: Health Claims for Soy Protein, Questions about Other Components," author John Henkel pinpoints the various health benefits of soy in the diet, stating that soy is a good substitute for animal protein because it is a complete protein, containing all the amino acids humans require without high levels of saturated fats. Referring to earlier studies, the author also notes that research suggests that soy proteins may lower the bad cholesterol levels in blood without affecting good cholesterol levels. In addition, eating soy may reduce the incidence of osteoporosis and certain cancers—studies were underway to determine soy's efficacy in these conditions.

However, in late 2017, the FDA proposed revoking its 1999 ruling and removing the authorized health claims for soy protein regarding heart disease. This proposal cites numerous studies published since 1999 that show inconsistent findings on the relationship between soy protein and heart disease, specifically soy's ability to lower low-density lipoprotein (LDL) cholesterol. While removing the authorized health claims, the proposal does recommend allowing qualified health claims if sufficient evidence supports a link between consuming soy protein and a reduced risk of heart disease. It's worth noting that the proposed rule does not address any of the other purported health benefits of soy, and the *Dietary Guidelines for Americans 2015–2020* do allow soy beverages and soy-protein products as part of a healthy eating pattern.

Additionally, following the FDA's 1999 endorsement of soy and its possible benefits, the American Heart Association issued an advisory recommending soy products, with their polyunsaturated fats and fiber and low saturated fat, as possibly beneficial as a source of protein. However, after reviewing twenty-two studies published after issuing its recommendation, the American Heart Association's Nutrition Committee slightly revised its earlier statement about soy intake and its relationship to heart disease. Its conclusion: soy protein reduced harmful cholesterol by only 3 percent and had virtually no effect on lowering blood pressure. The committee's report added that the findings on soy protein's worth in preventing or treating breast or prostate cancers is not established. But researchers did note that using various soy products with their polyunsaturated fats to replace high-fat proteins had dietary benefit.

The Health Risks of Soy

On the other side of the soy debate, soy detractors point out that eating soy not only has drawbacks; it also could have serious health effects. Some consumers have claimed that soy in infant formulas lowers IQ; others say soy causes thyroid problems.

The FDA itself in its 2000 article on soy confirmed that the jury may still be out for much of soy's touted health claims, particularly relating to soy isoflavones, which are a weak form of estrogen and in high levels could increase the risk of breast cancer. However, a study published by the *Cancer Project News* in 2006 that was conducted by the Johns Hopkins School of Medicine found that high soy intake actually reduced breast cancer risk, particularly for premenopausal women.

An additional soy detractor is the DC-based Weston A. Price Foundation, which has filed a petition with the FDA asking the government agency to amend its earlier pro-soy statements. The petition suggests that soy may play a role in promoting certain cancers, in initiating thyroid diseases, and causing reproductive problems. It cites that the to-date scientific findings about soy's health benefits are inconclusive. For more information, visit www.westonaprice.org.

Many people report allergic reactions to soy proteins, a fact substantiated by the Asthma and Allergy Foundation of America, which reports that soy is one of the most common allergens on the market. It also notes that not all soyfoods cause a reaction, but since soy is now prevalent in many food products, even if the label does not state that soy is present, avoiding soy is a challenge for the allergy sufferer.

Feeling Full on the Vegan Diet

If you are used to eating a heavier, meatier diet you may find yourself struggling with hunger when eating vegan. Remember, the vegan diet is not a calorie-restricting diet, so the solution, of course, is simple. If you are hungry, it means you aren't getting enough calories. Eat more!

If you're eating full, nutritionally balanced meals, it's unlikely that you'll experience this, but if you do find yourself constantly hungry or losing too much weight, opt for heavier foods, such as nuts, avocados, and meat substitutes, and fill up on fiber to help you feel full. Beans, lentils, and whole grains are a good source.

Vegan foods tend to be lower in calories than nonvegan foods, which means you may need to eat larger meals than you may be accustomed to. For example, 3 ounces of lean cooked beef has more than 150 calories, while 3 ounces of tofu has only 60 calories. You could eat two servings of tofu and still be consuming fewer calories than the beef! If you're hungry, fill up your plate with more food.

Hunger versus Food Cravings

Even though there's no reason to ever go hungry on a vegan diet, you may find yourself longing for specific foods. What's the difference between hunger and a food craving? If you're truly hungry, you'll eat just about anything to fill that physical void. But when you're craving a particular food, you're not actually hungry but are usually trying to fill an emotional void with a particular comforting taste. The easiest way to distinguish between the two is to ask yourself: "Would I want to eat an apple right now? Or a green salad?" If the answer is yes, then you're probably genuinely hungry. But if the answer is no, because all you really want is some ice cream or chocolate, then you're experiencing a food craving.

Cravings are a normal part of life, no matter what diet you follow! Dealing with them on the vegan diet may be as simple as finding a vegan substitute for whatever it is you're craving, or it may mean getting a bit creative. Go ahead and indulge in some vegan junk food from time to time, if that's really what you need in order to keep you on the healthy path in the long run. Ice cream, potato chips, cookies, and chocolate all have vegan versions that are readily available. Just make sure it's an occasional indulgence and not a daily habit.

Creative Ways to Satisfy Cravings

Even though a craving may seem to be for a particular food, it may actually be for a particular flavor or texture. A craving for sweet and sour chicken, for example, is mostly about the tangy sauce rather than the chicken itself. Why not cook up a chicken substitute or even tofu or tempeh in the same familiar sauce?

Vegan substitutes can be more satisfying than you might think. Taste works in combination with all of the other senses. The visual presentation, the texture, the feel of the food in our mouth, the smell, and even the sound a food makes as we chew it changes how we perceive it to taste. This is why it's so easy for vegan foods to substitute for the real thing. Take tofu scramble, for example. A good vegan scramble has tofu that is crumbled to resemble scrambled eggs, and it also has a bit of yellow coloring added to it with turmeric, curry powder, or nutritional yeast. Some recipes even call for black salt, which gives it an "eggy" smell. All of these elements fool your brain into thinking it's eating eggs while being perfectly satisfied with tofu. So go ahead, try a few substitutes with an open mind and make your transition just a little bit easier.

Hydration

One of the best ways to prevent pesky food cravings is to stay hydrated. It's common knowledge that staying hydrated has a multitude of benefits for your health, and one of these benefits is to keep you feeling full. If you're feeling hungry yet you've eaten sufficient calories, it may not be food your body needs but water. But how to make sure you've had enough? Though some nutritionists disagree that we all need 8 ounces, eight times a day, this gold standard is a good goal when changing your diet and trying to increase your health.

Bring a water bottle with you wherever you go and keep it filled up. Get in the habit of drinking a large glass of water first thing in the morning. It'll help wake you up and get your digestive system moving in the right direction to start the day. Just guzzle it down—no sipping! If you also drink a glass of water before each meal and snack, you're well on your way to meeting your hydration needs. Another idea is to fill up a pitcher of water with two quarts (a little less than two liters) of water and make sure that you drink it all throughout the day. If you're not used to drinking so much water, you may find for the first couple days that you need to urinate more frequently, but your body will soon adjust, and you'll be rewarded with more energy, better skin, enhanced digestion, and better overall health.

Bloating

As your body adjusts to a vegan diet, you may experience a bit of bloating. Although it's not often talked about, there's also the possibility of a bit of extra gas. Not everyone experiences this, but it can certainly be discouraging if you do! You can prevent bloating and gas before they even happen by drinking plenty of water. If you're cooking beans from scratch, make sure they're fully cooked and switch out the soaking water with fresh water before cooking. When using canned beans, draining and rinsing them well helps rid the beans of the sugars that produce gas. Another culprit may be too much processed meat substitutes or even too much soy milk. Try sticking to simpler meals with fewer mock meats and switching to almond milk until your body adjusts to your new diet. Ease back into the offending foods slowly, with small portions to start.

5

Ingredients for Healthy Vegan Cooking

Make friends with your kitchen. As with any kitchen setting, the vegan kitchen—even if you are the only one in the household on a plant-based diet—needs some adjusting. For example, your pantry may need a makeover that's more veg-friendly.

This doesn't mean that you have to discard what other family members choose to eat. If your partner or children still enjoy their chicken cutlets, for example, keep them in the freezer, but make room for what's important to you.

This chapter will help you stock your shelves with ingredients that will make cooking for the vegan diet quick, easy, and delicious. You'll also find some tips for working with vegan ingredients like tofu and easy ways to adapt your favorite recipes to fit the vegan diet.

Basic Pantry Items

This is really about going back to the basics. Think about those possible meals when you will be too tired or too rushed to slow cook a grains-based meal. That's when you'll miss out on some good eating, especially if you don't have your pantry stocked with such basics as canned beans, already made vegetable broth and soups, and plenty of dried herbs. Such staples are handy when you run out of time and energy but still want a tasty meal.

You can also stock up on aseptically packaged tofu and soy milk, sealed packets of seaweed to top your miso soup, handy prepacked soup mixes, energy bars, and even a good supply of ready-to-eat nuts and seeds. Some markets also sell precooked and vacuum-packed brown and wild rice and noodles. So, look at your cupboards, rethink your eating plans, then make your pantry and fridge fit into your lifestyle. Don't forget about filling your freezer with ready-made vegan or vegetarian entrées and "burgers." Most major brands produce some vegan or vegetarian products, so scout out the freezer cases.

Other Vegan Staples

Like to experiment with ethnic dishes but don't have time to race around town regularly? Take several hours of your free time some weekend and stock up on loads of basics. At an Indian grocery you'll find lentils of every color, to say nothing of a slew of exotic spices. Hispanic markets are good sources for dried beans of many different varieties, and often these come in economy-sized bags for budget-conscious shoppers.

Love Asian noodles? Asian markets will seem like a treasure chest, for you can pick up dried noodles from China, Vietnam, Japan, and Thailand in one stop. You may even find seasoning staples such as fresh lemongrass, assorted makes of canned coconut milk, and seasoning pastes and sauces to suit every palate. If you plan to cook within a few days after shopping, bring home some of the fresh noodle varieties and add to your basket some of the assorted fresh tofu products.

Sugars versus Natural Sweeteners

Some manufacturers produce granulated sugars by filtering raw cane sugars through charred animal bones. It's impossible for consumers to know how the sugar is produced, so vegans often turn to other natural sweeteners. Strict vegans also won't sweeten foods with honey because it is the product of living creatures.

Whether or not you omit these sweeteners from your pantry doesn't mean you can't add a dash of something sweet to your pan. Agave nectar, date sugar, maple syrup, and stevia are perfectly sweet and perfectly acceptable.

Oils, Fats, and Nonstick Cooking Sprays

In place of butter, select a good nonhydrogenated margarine, one that does not contain the animal product whey. Some vegan cooks replace fat in baking with such ingredients as applesauce and mashed bananas.

With all the fuss about trans fats, hydrogenated fats, and heart health, picking out what's healthiest is important. Every diet should include some oils, and you should keep quality olive oils—preferably extra-virgin oils for heightening flavors, though not really for cooking—on hand. Specialty oils useful for adding a flavor profile include toasted sesame oil, hazelnut oil, and walnut oil.

But the trick is to keep fat intake down, even if your fat source is a so-called healthy oil.

You should also select a good quality vegetable oil, such as peanut or canola oil, for your sautéing and stir-frying.

To slash the fat in the many vegan recipes that call for sautéing onions, garlic, or veggies in oil, use half oil and half vegetable broth; soy sauce; or even cooking wine, sherry, or another liquid. Some chefs call this technique "steam-frying."

And if you really are looking to trim fats, keep a container on hand of nonstick cooking spray: this could become indispensable for any quick panfrying you do.

Flours

The next time you browse the baking aisle, check out the many types of flours on sale: the options may seem bewildering—from pastry flours to self-rising flours to cake flours to the general all-purpose types. So, here's your chance to know ahead what is in the bag. For general all-purpose baking, the all-purpose white flours are fine, but look for a brand that at least is unbleached and, better yet, also contains flour from organic wheat or other grains.

Whole-wheat flours are fine for sturdier baked goods, but they don't produce as fine a crumb and are not really suitable for delicate pastries. Yet because these flours still contain the whole bran and wheat germ, they contain more nutrients. Relatively new to the marketplace are the white whole-wheat flours, which contain all the nutrients and fiber of whole-wheat flours but bake up like pastry flours. Several manufacturers retail this product made from organically grown wheats, a double benefit for the consumer.

Egg Substitutes

Health-food stores, high-end grocery stores, and many regular grocery stores now sell packaged egg replacements, such as Ener-G Egg Replacer and Orgran No Egg Natural Egg Replacer. These products are convenient and easy to use! For most recipes, follow the directions on the box to combine the appropriate amounts of egg replacer and water and allow to sit for a few minutes to thicken before adding to the rest of the ingredients.

Baking Soda and Vinegar

1 egg = 1 teaspoon baking soda + 1 tablespoon vinegar

When eggs are used as a leavening agent, a combination of baking soda and vinegar can do the trick!

The chemical reaction that occurs when baking soda is mixed with vinegar causes the release of bubbles of carbon dioxide gas, which works great for providing lift to a cake or cupcake batter. The baking soda and vinegar mixture often works best when gently stirred into the batter as the final ingredient. The reaction will start right away, so be careful not to stir the batter any more than needed, or too many of the gas bubbles will burst and the cake won't rise! Once mixed, the batter should then be quickly poured into the desired pans or cupcake tins and immediately placed in the preheated oven to bake according to the recipe directions. Use either white distilled vinegar or apple cider vinegar.

Flaxseeds

1 egg = 1 tablespoon ground flaxseeds + 3 tablespoons water

Flaxseeds become quite thick and gooey when ground into a meal and mixed with water. Flaxseeds will add a nutty flavor, and the ground-up bits may be visible in the finished product, so they may be best used in heartier recipes, such as whole-wheat bread.

Silken Tofu

1 egg = ¼ cup silken tofu

For quiches and fillings, such as puddings, curds, cheesecake, and custards, silken tofu is a wonderful substitute for eggs! Tofu should be well drained and wiped off with paper towels to remove any excess moisture before being blended for your recipe.

Bananas and Applesauce

Just as these fruits are good fat replacers, they also function pretty well as egg replacers in sweet recipes. Add an extra ½ teaspoon of baking powder to your recipe to help keep the texture of the baked good lighter. For 1 egg, mash ½ of a ripe banana or use ¼ cup applesauce.

Dairy Substitutes

When it comes to shopping for vegan dairy products today, there have never been more choices! Dairy products such as milk serve to contribute flavor and moisture to baked goods. Other dairy products used in baking include cream, nonfat dry milk powder, sour cream, cream cheese, yogurt, evaporated milk, sweetened condensed milk, and buttermilk.

Milk

Milk can be replaced with any number of alternatives, such as soy, almond, hemp, rice, and coconut milks; however, soy milk is the most similar in protein content and other nutrients and will perform more like milk than other substitutes. Rice milk is thinner and sweeter than soy milk, and almond milk has a grainier texture. For baking, soy or almond milk is best, and in savory casseroles and sauces, use soy milk for its neutral flavor. Choose brands fortified with vitamin D, B_{12}, and calcium, particularly if you've got kids.

Cream or Half-and-Half

Nondairy creamers, such as Silk and Organic Valley brands, are thick and rich, making them a fantastic substitute for cream!

Nonfat Dry Milk Powder

There are two options for replacing nonfat dry milk powder in your recipes. First of all, you can purchase a can of soy milk powder, such as the brand Better Than Milk. Use it in the recipe as you would the nonfat dry milk powder. The second option is to first calculate the amount of milk that would be reconstituted from the amount of nonfat dry milk powder required by the recipe and then replace that amount of liquid from the recipe with the same amount of soy milk. Since the ratio of nonfat dry milk powder to water is usually 1 to 4, if a recipe called for 1 tablespoon of nonfat dry milk powder, that would mean that you would need 4 tablespoons or ¼ cup of water to reconstitute that milk. So, you would reduce the amount of liquid in your recipe by ¼ cup and add the ¼ cup soy milk.

Sour Cream and Cream Cheese

Sour cream is easily replaced with a vegan sour cream. Tofutti has a delicious, cool, and creamy sour cream called Sour Supreme. Tofutti also offers a good cream cheese substitute called Better Than Cream Cheese.

Yogurt

There are a variety of soy and other nondairy yogurts on the market these days. Look for brands that contain live cultures! As with replacing milk with soy milk, soy yogurt is likely to more closely resemble the nutrition profile of dairy yogurt than some of the other nondairy yogurt options.

Evaporated Milk and Sweetened Condensed Milk

Evaporated milk is like taking 1 cup of water and adding twice as much dry milk powder as needed to make 1 cup of milk. In other words, it's double strength! To make 1 cup of vegan evaporated milk, simply measure 1 cup of water and add two times the soy milk powder needed to make 1 cup of regular-strength soy milk.

For sweetened condensed milk, make 1 cup of vegan evaporated milk, as described above. Then add 1½ cups sugar and stir over medium heat until sugar is dissolved.

Buttermilk

Buttermilk's functions in baking are very important! First of all, buttermilk contributes to leavening. Buttermilk is acidic, and when mixed into a recipe along with baking soda or baking powder, the acid of the buttermilk will react with the alkalinity of the baking soda or baking powder, producing the carbon dioxide bubbles that help baked goods rise. Buttermilk also adds flavor. To make 1 cup of vegan buttermilk, place 1 tablespoon of vinegar or lemon juice in the bottom of a measuring cup. Add enough soy milk to make 1 cup. Stir and allow to thicken or "curdle" for 10–15 minutes. Your "buttermilk" is now ready to use!

Breads, Baked Goods, and Pastas

Finding vegan bread and baked goods in a supermarket can be challenging. Many breads contain whey (a milk derivative), eggs, or honey. Rye breads often appear to be vegan, and some traditional French or Italian breads are vegan as well. You may have better luck at a store with a natural foods or ethnic section.

Many brands of pasta are vegan. Some will have eggs added, especially noodles or fettuccine, so check the label. Pasta sauces may have meat or cheese added; marinara sauces are often vegan.

Food Labeling

It's become most people's habit to read food labels, especially to figure out the calorie counts; fat grams; amounts of added sugars, such as sucrose, fructose, or glucose; and the amounts of sodium. Sodium levels can be particularly high with canned beans, and even if you like using the liquid packed with the beans, you'd be better off draining and rinsing the beans—and getting rid of excess sodium—before you use them.

As you look for whole-grain items, be sure that the word "whole-grain" comes first or second on the ingredients list; otherwise, you may be getting a product that is not as wholesome as you want.

If you do stock up on canned goods, you should check that the products you buy are as free of added chemicals and preservatives as possible. You'll also want to wise up on the number of servings and the calorie counts per serving—nutrition labels tell you what you find in one serving only—do not make the mistake that the figures refer to the entire contents.

The Whys of Vegan and Vegetarian Labeling

When shopping, you must also learn to check the fine print: some manufacturers may disguise the fact that their product contains some animal product or products. Such ingredients as casein, rennet, gelatin, and glycerides all come from animals.

As the Vegetarian Resource Group points out, retailers now often package their vegetarian products with a vegetarian or vegan symbol. Finding such a symbol or all-veg food label should reassure you that what you are buying is free of animal products, but there are no federal rules regulating the use of "vegan" on labels. Some private companies and nonprofit organizations have developed their own standards and guidelines as to what a vegan food is. To determine if a food meets your definition of vegan, check the ingredient listing.

If an ingredient listing contains the term "natural flavors," the USDA's Food Safety and Inspection Service (FSIS) requires that if the natural flavors are derived from animal sources, the label indicates this. The term "natural flavors" on a label without additional qualification means spices, spice extracts, or essential oils were used to flavor the food. Some obvious signs that a food isn't vegan are meat, fish, poultry, egg, or dairy ingredients. Then there are ingredients like gelatin, beef broth, lard, and Worcestershire sauce (contains anchovies) that are derived from meat or fish. Dairy-derived ingredients include casein (milk protein), whey, and lactase (milk sugar). Some ingredients sound like they might be dairy derived but aren't, like cocoa butter, cream of tartar, and lactic acid.

Shopping Tips

Health-food stores and gourmet grocers stock vegan specialty goods, but these days even most regular chain supermarkets carry mock meats and dairy substitutes. Some stores have a separate "natural foods" aisle, while others stock the veggie burgers with the other frozen foods. Most health-food stores and co-ops are happy to place special orders, so don't be afraid to ask.

Browse farmers' markets and farm stands for good deals. Community-supported agriculture, or CSAs, provide a way for the consumer to buy into, or subscribe to, a farmer's weekly production of vegetables, fruits, and other farm goods. This benefits both the farmer, who is assured of selling what he grows, and the consumer, who gets weekly deliveries of farm-fresh goods. Most areas of the country have nearby farmers who participate in a CSA.

Seek out ethnic and import grocers for hidden treasures. Kosher stores stock enough dairy substitutes to fill a vegan's dreams; Asian grocery stores are a paradise of exotic meatless "meats," sauces, and spices; and Middle Eastern and Mexican grocers supply unusual ingredients and flavors.

Insiders know that the Seventh-day Adventist religion has a long history of vegetarianism and even their own brand of veggie "meats." Check out Adventist book supply stores for a bounty of veggie hams, fish, and sausages if you're lucky enough to have one in your area!

Vegan Foods in a Grocery Store

The grocery section is one part of the store where you can find items you never real-ized were vegan. It's worthwhile to occasionally spend an hour or so in this section, reading labels and making notes of unexpected "finds." Here are some tips for ap-proaching this section of the store:

- If you're looking for a cracker, steer clear of those with cheese or butter in the product's name. Crackers with whole-wheat flour as the first ingredient are a bet-ter choice than those with wheat flour listed first.
- Many canned fruits, beans, and vegetables are vegan. Check vegetable labels for added salt pork, bacon, or other meat ingredients. These are especially common in canned greens and beans.
- Hot cereals like oatmeal, grits, and polenta are often vegan. Often the plain (or original) version will simply have the grain as its ingredient. Check the labels on hot cereals for milk or cheese.
- The ethnic section of the grocery store can have some interesting items. Look for falafel mix in the Middle Eastern section, lard-free refried beans in the Hispanic section, and unusual dried noodles in the Asian section.
- Some supermarkets also have a natural foods section. Of course, all items are not vegan, but this may be where you will find aseptically packaged soy milk, vegan canned soups, and vegan breakfast cereals.
- While not the healthiest part of the store, the snacks aisle does include vegan potato chips, pretzels, tortilla chips, and other munchables. Watch for added cheese or other dairy products.

Frozen Foods

The frozen foods section is where you'll find frozen vegetables (great for times when the produce drawer is empty and your dinner needs a vegetable), frozen fruits (think smoothies), frozen juice concentrate, and frequently frozen veggie burgers. There may be other surprises like vegan pierogi, vegan soups, and vegan frozen desserts.

Are frozen vegetables more nutritious than fresh? It depends. Frozen vegetables are frequently processed immediately after they're picked to minimize nutrient loss. After harvesting, vegetables lose vitamins with exposure to air and sunlight. So, if the fresh broccoli is several days away from when it was picked, it may be significantly lower in some vitamins than frozen broccoli.

Staples to Stock

Sensible cooks of every persuasion stock their cupboards—and refrigerator and freezer—with some handy items, not only for use in emergency situations but also for everyday cooking. Some examples include:

Dry Goods

- Baking powder, baking soda, and cornstarch
- Rice, including long-grain white rice, such as jasmine or basmati, and brown rice
- Legumes, such as canned and dried beans, split peas, and lentils
- Whole grains, including cracked wheat, cornmeal, and quinoa
- Flours
- Sweeteners
- Pastas, both dried and fresh
- Hot and cold cereals

Condiments and Seasonings

- Soy sauce; low-sodium soy sauce is a healthful choice
- Vinegars, such as balsamic, white, and herbed
- Extracts, including vanilla, lemon, and almond extracts
- Herbs such as dried oregano, dried thyme, ground turmeric, and ground cumin
- Spices such as ground cinnamon and cinnamon sticks, ground nutmeg, ground cloves, and ground ginger
- Ketchup, mustard, and vegan mayonnaise
- Pickles and relishes
- Beverages, including tea leaves, coffee beans, and fruit juices; also, keep handy soy milks in shelf-stable cartons
- Oils, including olive oil and canola oil

For the Refrigerator

- Nut butters
- Tofu of varying textures

- Tempeh
- Vegan dairy-replacement foods, such as vegan cheese and vegan margarine

Although some of these items are perishable, they are handy in a pinch.

For the Freezer

- Frozen cooked-ahead meals
- Boxes of frozen vegetables
- Commercial vegan breakfast and dinner entrées and pasta dishes

What you store away for future use can save you cooking headaches on those days when you have no free time for cooking.

Onions and Garlic

Favorite flavor enhancers, onions, garlic, scallions, and leeks—members of the Alliaceae family—have universal appeal. Onions come in many sizes and shapes, ranging from the small, white pearl onions to the round, red onions to the slightly flattened, golden-skinned Vidalia and the smaller Italian cipollini. These onions are "cured" so that the skin turns papery, protecting the onion interior from decay; these must be stored in cool, dry places, not in the refrigerator. The other stalklike onions—leeks and scallions, for example—are always fresh, with white bulbs and long, green leaves furled lengthwise; these fresh onions should be plastic-wrapped and refrigerated.

Fresh heads of garlic are readily available in supermarkets, and for added convenience, many manufacturers now sell pre-peeled garlic cloves, chopped garlic packed in oil, garlic pastes, garlic salt, and dried garlic flakes. But for the best flavors, it's hard to pass up the fresh heads in their papery coverings.

Be sure to select heads that are firm without any soft spots or green sprouts, both signs of garlic going bad. At home, store garlic in a cool, dry place, discarding any cloves that are beginning to soften. To cook with garlic, separate the cloves from the head pressing down on the whole head with your hand or with the flat side of a cleaver or other broad knife. Then peel the papery skins off each clove and crush or mince the garlic as desired.

Parsley

An essential herb, parsley in all its various guises—curly-leaf and flat-leaf—not only garnishes plates and a finished dish; it also adds its own characteristic flavor that ranges from mildly pungent to earthy-soapy, as some describe cilantro. Besides its uses in the kitchen, according to some research from the University of Kentucky, parsley also may offer several health benefits: it is an antioxidant, and it also may help prevent or deter certain cancers.

Although it is botanically a member of the carrot family, cilantro, also known as Chinese parsley, is used much the same way as standard parsley: as a garnish and as a flavor booster. The leaves of the coriander plant, cilantro is a must-have seasoning in many Hispanic, Caribbean, Asian, and Indian dishes; many North American cooks, too, have come to appreciate its pungent-acidic-earthy taste. Of course, whole or ground coriander seeds are mainstays of many international kitchens.

The Basils

Considered by many as the king of herbs, basil in all its forms—from the richly scented Thai basils to the sweet basils such as lemon basil, cinnamon basil, and Genovese basil—is an annual that is easy to grow and, fortunately, is available year-round in most supermarkets; some varieties are classed as tender perennials. Beloved for its minty fragrance and flavor accent, the basils also contain essential oils that may figure in reducing inflammation, fighting certain bacteria, and even promoting heart health.

Tarragon, Dill, Oregano, and Thyme

Strongly flavored, these herbs play critical roles in seasoning savory dishes, but all should be used sparingly until you find your comfort level with their flavors. Tarragon, with its unmistakable minty taste, plays a key role in French cooking and is used often in herb blends. Dill, or dill weed, is a parsley relative. Its fresh feathery leaves highlight breads, salads, and cheese, but because its leaves are heat sensitive, dill should be added to hot dishes just before serving; its seeds are favored for pickling and in salad dressings. Hailing originally from the Mediterranean region, oregano is popular world-wide for its earthy aroma that accents every kind of ingredient. Thyme has a warm yet delicate taste that heightens the flavors of many vegetarian dishes.

Mint

A many-splendored and many-faceted herb with a lively and complex flavor, mint in its many guises suits both sweet and savory dishes, and mint makes an elegant addition to a variety of beverages, including Kentucky's famed mint julep. Most mints are easy-to-grow perennials and, with careful tending, spread prolifically.

You should try to use fresh herbs whenever possible; dried herbs lose potency quickly and must be used sparingly. Dried herbs also produce a much more intense flavor because their natural oils have become concentrated. If you are using them dried, check the herbs before seasoning: if their aroma seems musty or their color has turned grayish, they are probably past their potency, and you should discard them.

Vegan Substitution Chart

Once you know a thing or two about some common vegan substitutes, veganizing your favorite recipes is easy. With a little know-how, you can find a reasonable stand-in for just about any ingredient you need, and you can make the same cookies, cakes, and muffins you've always enjoyed with egg and dairy substitutes. Most larger grocery stores stock several vegan substitute products, but for greater variety, stop by any natural foods store.

Vegan Substitution Chart		
Instead of this:	**Use this:**	**Notes:**
Butter	Vegan margarine, soy margarine	Vegan margarine works just fine in baked goods, sauces, and just about everything. One popular brand is Earth Balance.
Milk	Soy milk, almond milk, or rice milk	Rice milk is thinner and sweeter, with less fat. Stick with soy or almond for savory dishes and baking. Rice milk works best in smoothies and with breakfast cereals.
Cream	Soy cream, coconut cream	
Parmesan cheese	Nutritional yeast or Parmesan cheese substitute (try Parma brand)	
Egg	Store-bought egg replacer (try Ener-G or Bob's Red Mill brand), 1 tablespoon flax meal mixed with 3 tablespoons water, ¼ cup applesauce	These egg substitutes work great in baked goods such as cookies, muffins, and cakes.

Mayonnaise	Store-bought vegan mayonnaise, homemade vegan mayonnaise, hummus, or pesto	Vegan mayonnaise is quite tasty, but try expanding your horizons on sandwiches with different spreads, whether homemade or store-bought.
Buttermilk	1 tablespoon lemon juice or vinegar mixed with 1 cup unsweetened soy milk	It's not quite as thick, but the acidity of the lemon juice or vinegar provides tanginess similar to buttermilk.
Cheese	Nondairy vegan cheese made from soy, rice, or almonds	Vegan Gourmet, Daiya, and Teese are the most popular brands, but there are several on the market to choose from. Watch out for casein (milk protein) in other brands. Alternatives exist for everything from mozzarella to feta.
Chocolate	Vegan chocolate	Many chocolate bars and chocolate chips are dairy-free. Just skim the ingredients list or look for brands labeled as vegan.
Yogurt	Soy yogurt	Try Silk brand. Check the dairy section of your grocery store.
Fish sauce	Soy sauce with a squeeze of lime	A common ingredient in Thai cuisine, vegetarian fish sauce is also available at some Asian grocers.
Oyster Sauce	Vegetarian oyster sauce	Another ingredient common in Asian meals, the vegetarian version is made from mushrooms and is standard in ethnic food aisles.

Honey	Agave nectar	Agave has a similar taste and consistency to honey, making it the perfect substitute.
Meat-based stocks, chicken broth	Vegetable broth, vegetarian bouillon	Watch out for monosodium glutamate (MSG) in bouillon and powdered vegetable broth.

Basic Cooking Techniques

Here is a list of basic cooking methods and a description of each one:

Stir-frying: The traditional Chinese cooking method calls for quick cooking cut-up foods in a little oil over high heat while you constantly stir and toss the ingredients. Cook the densest vegetables first, the most delicate last. Correct stir-frying retains both the texture and flavor of the ingredient.

Sautéing: Similar to stir-frying, sautéing quick-cooks foods in minimal amounts of oil; this is useful for larger cuts of vegetables.

Roasting: Oven-roasting vegetables is a popular and effective way to slow cook batches of whole or cut-up vegetables, either alone or combined with other varieties. To prevent drying out, vegetables should be tossed in minimal amounts of oil; flavoring the vegetables with herbs and other seasonings yields delectable results. This slow-cooking method draws out natural flavors.

Poaching: A low-fat way to cook vegetables, poaching calls for cooking a vegetable in a small amount of water or vegetable broth; you can season the cooking liquid with herbs if you want. For uniform cooking, the vegetable or vegetables should be cut to similar sizes.

Steaming: Adherents of steaming vegetables point out that this slow-cooking method in which the vegetable sits above, not in, the cooking water retains nutrients and produces a crisp-tender result. The trick is keeping the steaming basket above the boiling water and covering the slow cooker so steam does not escape.

Blanching vegetables: Blanching helps retain natural color lost in high-heat cooking. Just plunge vegetables into boiling water for several seconds and then plunge into ice water to stop the cooking. The outer layers soften without losing crispness. You can use blanched vegetables in salads and other cold dishes, add them to stews or soups, or finish cooking them in a stir-fry.

Make Your Favorite Recipes Vegan

When you start a vegan diet, there's no need to toss out all your old cookbooks and family recipes. Many of them can provide inspiration for fabulous vegan meals after a few minor tweaks, of course. Most recipes for cookies, muffins, and cakes can be made with nondairy milk, vegan margarine, and a commercial egg replacer. For recipes calling for honey, try an equivalent amount of agave nectar, which is equally lovely in tea and drizzled over vegan pancakes. Store-bought mock ground beef is surprisingly tasty, TVP granules provide a meaty texture in dishes such as tacos or chili.

Take a look at some of your favorite meals. Do you like spaghetti with meatballs? Try a vegetable marinara instead or grab some ready-made vegetarian meatballs from your grocery store. You can make your favorite chicken noodle soup recipe without the chicken and omit the beef from your Chinese beef and broccoli, or use seitan as a beef substitute instead. Often, it's the spices, flavors, and textures that make a meal satisfying and nostalgic, not the actual meat.

For the novice chef, restaurants can offer a tasty introduction to new foods. Search online for vegan restaurants in your area. Thai and Chinese restaurants serve up vegan curries and stir-fries, many with an array of mock meats. As a general rule, ethnic restaurants including Mexican (just hold the cheese), Indian, and Middle Eastern places provide more options for vegetarians and vegans than American chains and diners, which may offer little more than a veggie burger as an afterthought.

Vegan Mashed Potato Tricks

There's nothing wrong with just switching the butter and milk for vegan versions in your favorite potato recipe, but half a container of nondairy sour cream or cream cheese, a few teaspoons of fresh crumbled sage, or some chopped artichoke hearts will make your spuds come alive. Or simply add a shake of nutmeg or rosemary.

Varieties of Veggie Broths

A basic vegetable broth is made by simmering vegetables, potatoes, and a bay leaf or two in water for at least 30 minutes. While you may be familiar with the canned and boxed stocks available at the grocery store, vegan chefs have a few other tricks up their sleeves to impart extra flavor to recipes calling for vegetable broth. Check your natural grocer for specialty flavored bouillon cubes such as vegetarian "chicken" or "beef" flavor or shop the bulk bins for powdered vegetable broth mix.

Dried versus Canned Beans

Canned beans are convenient, but dried beans are cheaper, use less packaging, and add a fresher flavor. And if you plan in advance, they aren't much work at all to prepare. Place beans in a large pot, cover with water (more than you think you'll need), and allow to sit for at least 2 hours or overnight. Drain the water and simmer in fresh water for about an hour, then you're good to go! One cup of dried beans yields about 3 cups cooked.

Easy Vegan Seasoning Blend

Garlic powder, nutritional yeast, and salt is a delicious seasoning combination and will give you a bit of a B_{12} perk-up. Use it over toast, veggies, popcorn, bagels, baked potatoes, and, of course, cooked pasta if you're feeling, well, lazy and hungry!

Basic Vegan White Sauce

Melted vegan margarine, along with soy milk, is the base for many vegan cream sauces, roux, and cheese sauces. Flour is the simplest thickener, but cornstarch or arrowroot also works. Nutritional yeast is added for a cheesy flavor, and garlic powder, onion powder, and salt enhance the general flavor. Use an unsweetened soy milk for a more savory taste.

Pressing and Freezing Tofu

Tofu doesn't taste like much on its own, but it soaks up spices and marinades wonderfully.

It's like a sponge: the drier it is, the more flavor it absorbs. Wrap firm tofu in a couple layers of paper towels and place a can of beans or another light weight on top. After 10 minutes, flip the tofu over and let it sit weighted down for another 10 minutes. "Pressing" firm and extra-firm tofu will substantially enhance just about every recipe.

Freezing firm or extra-firm tofu creates an even meatier and chewier texture, which some people prefer, and makes it even more absorbent. After pressing your tofu, stick it in the freezer until solid and thaw just before using. If you don't use the whole block, cover any leftover bits of uncooked tofu with water in a sealed container and stick it in the fridge.

Marinating Tofu

For marinated baked tofu dishes, a zip-top bag can be helpful in getting the tofu well covered with marinade. Place the tofu in the bag, pour the marinade in, seal, and set in the fridge, turning and lightly shaking occasionally to coat all sides of the tofu.

Cleaning a Portobello Mushroom

As with any mushroom variety, portobellos do not need rinsing, rather a simple wipe-off with a moist paper towel. Then carefully twist off the mushroom's stem. You may also want to remove the black gills under the cap. To do this, use a spoon and gently scrape them away. The gills impart a dark color to any surrounding liquids.

6

50+ Recipes for Your Vegan Diet

The vegan diet is full of fresh ingredients and delicious flavors. In this chapter you'll find a range of recipes to help you get started with the vegan diet. Many are vegan takes on classic favorites including Super "Meaty" Chili with TVP, Dairy-Free Ranch Dressing, Potatoes "Au Gratin" Casserole, and Breaded Eggplant "Parmesan." From breakfasts to dinner with soups, salads, and snacks in between, every meal is covered. And of course, there's always room for desserts like Strawberry Coconut Ice Cream and Classic Chocolate Chip Cookies.

Super Green Quiche

Get your greens in before noon with this veggie quiche. To avoid a crumbly mess, you'll have to be patient and let it cool before slicing.

Serves 4

1 (10-ounce) package frozen chopped spinach, thawed and drained
½ cup broccoli, diced small
1 (12-ounce) block firm or extra-firm tofu
1 tablespoon soy sauce
¼ cup soy milk
1 teaspoon mustard

2 tablespoons nutritional yeast
½ teaspoon garlic powder
1 teaspoon parsley
½ teaspoon rosemary
¾ teaspoon salt
¼ teaspoon pepper
Prepared vegan crust (see sidebar)

1. Preheat oven to 350°F.
2. Place the spinach and broccoli in a steamer basket over boiling water until just lightly cooked, then set aside to cool. Press as much moisture as possible out of the spinach.
3. In a blender or food processor, combine the tofu with the remaining ingredients, except crust, until well mixed. Mix in the spinach and broccoli by hand until combined.
4. Spread mixture evenly in prepared pie crust.
5. Bake for 35–40 minutes or until firm. Allow to cool for at least 10 minutes before serving. Quiche will firm up a bit more as it cools.

PER SERVING		
Calories: 326	Protein: 15 g	Carbohydrates: 24 g
Fat: 20 g	Sodium: 1,529 mg	Sugar: 2 g
	Fiber: 6 g	

An Easy Whole-Wheat Crust

Combine ¾ cup whole-wheat flour with ¾ cup all-purpose flour and a teaspoon of salt. Cut in ⅓ cup vegan margarine until it's crumbly, then add ice-cold water, a few tablespoons at a time, until you can form a dough. You'll need about ½ cup. Roll out the dough and press it into your pie pan and you're ready to fill it up!

Quick Tofu Breakfast Burrito

Toss in a fresh diced chili if you need something to really wake you up in the morning. There's no reason you can't enjoy these burritos for lunch either! Add ketchup or hot sauce for some extra flavor.

Serves 2

1 (12-ounce) block firm or extra-firm tofu, well pressed
2 tablespoons olive oil
½ cup salsa
½ teaspoon chili powder
¼ teaspoon salt
⅛ teaspoon pepper
2 (6") flour tortillas, warmed
2 slices vegan cheese
½ avocado, sliced

1. Cube or crumble the tofu into 1" chunks. Sauté in olive oil in large pan over medium heat for 2–3 minutes.
2. Add salsa and chili powder, and cook for 2–3 more minutes, stirring frequently. Season with salt and pepper.
3. Layer each warmed flour tortilla with half of the tofu and salsa mix and drizzle with ketchup or hot sauce.
4. Add vegan cheese and avocado slices and wrap like a burrito.

PER SERVING
Calories: 525
Fat: 38 g
Protein: 21 g
Sodium: 1,186 mg
Fiber: 8 g
Carbohydrates: 30 g
Sugar: 5 g

Easy Vegan French Toast

Kids love golden fried French toast drowning in powdered sugar and maple syrup, but a fruit compote or some agave nectar would be just as sweet.

Serves 4

2 medium bananas
½ cup soy milk
1 tablespoon orange juice
1 tablespoon maple syrup
¾ teaspoon vanilla

1 tablespoon flour
1 teaspoon cinnamon
½ teaspoon nutmeg
Oil or vegan margarine for frying
12 thick slices bread

1. Using a blender or mixer, mix together the bananas, soy milk, orange juice, maple syrup, and vanilla until smooth and creamy.
2. Whisk in flour, cinnamon, and nutmeg, and pour into a pie plate or shallow pan.
3. Heat 1–2 tablespoons of vegan margarine or oil in a large skillet.
4. Dip or spoon mixture over each bread slice on both sides and fry in hot oil until lightly golden brown on both sides, about 2–3 minutes.

PER SERVING			
Calories: 385	Fat: 9 g	Sodium: 518 mg	Carbohydrates: 66 g
	Protein: 10 g	Fiber: 5 g	Sugar: 17 g

Baked "Sausage" and Mushroom Frittata

Baked tofu frittatas are an easy brunch or weekend breakfast. Once you've got the technique down, it's easy to adjust the ingredients to your liking. With tofu and mock meat, this one packs a super protein punch!

Serves 4

½ medium yellow onion, diced
3 cloves garlic, minced
½ cup sliced mushrooms
1 (12-ounce) package vegetarian sausage
   substitute crumbles
2 tablespoons olive oil
¾ teaspoon salt

¼ teaspoon black pepper
1 (12-ounce) block firm or extra-firm tofu
1 (12-ounce) block silken tofu
1 tablespoon soy sauce
2 tablespoons nutritional yeast
¼ teaspoon turmeric
1 medium tomato, sliced thin

1. Preheat oven to 325°F and lightly grease a glass pie pan.
2. Heat onion, garlic, mushrooms, and vegetarian sausage in olive oil in a large skillet over medium heat for 3–4 minutes until sausage is browned and mushrooms are soft. Season with salt and pepper and set aside.
3. Combine firm tofu, silken tofu, soy sauce, nutritional yeast, and turmeric in a blender, and process until mixed. Combine tofu with sausage mixture and spread into pan. Layer slices of tomato on top.
4. Bake in oven for about 45 minutes or until firm. Allow to cool for 5–10 minutes before serving, as frittata will set as it cools.

PER SERVING	Fat: 15 g	Sodium: 1,059 mg	Carbohydrates: 16 g
Calories: 307	Protein: 31 g	Fiber: 6 g	Sugar: 4 g

Tofu Florentine

Satisfy your comfort food cravings with this "eggy" tofu and spinach mixture drowning in a creamy Quick Hollandaise Sauce on toast.

Serves 2

1 (12-ounce) block firm or extra-firm tofu, well pressed
2 tablespoons flour
1 teaspoon nutritional yeast
1 teaspoon garlic powder
2 tablespoons canola or safflower oil

1 (10-ounce) box frozen spinach, thawed and drained
½ cup Quick Hollandaise Sauce (see sidebar), divided
2 slices whole-wheat bread, lightly toasted

1. Slice tofu into ½"-thick slabs.
2. In a small bowl, combine the flour, nutritional yeast, and garlic powder. Dredge tofu in this mixture, then fry in oil for 2–3 minutes on each side until lightly browned.
3. Reduce heat and add spinach and 2 tablespoons of hollandaise sauce, gently coating tofu. Cook for just a minute or 2 over low heat until spinach is heated through.
4. Stack spinach and 2 strips of tofu mixture on each piece of toasted bread and cover with remaining sauce.

PER SERVING	Fat: 39 g	Sodium: 1,358 mg	Carbohydrates: 35 g
Calories: 599	Protein: 26 g	Fiber: 9 g	Sugar: 4 g

Quick Hollandaise Sauce

Makes ½ cup sauce

⅓ cup vegan mayonnaise
¼ cup lemon juice
3 tablespoons unsweetened soy milk
1½ tablespoons Dijon mustard
¼ teaspoon turmeric
½ teaspoon salt
¼ teaspoon black pepper
Whisk together all ingredients and heat over low heat before serving.
Adjust seasonings to taste.

Whole-Wheat Blueberry Muffins

Because these muffins have very little fat, they'll want to stick to the papers or the muffin tin. Letting them cool before removing them will help prevent this, and be sure to grease your muffin tin well.

Makes 18 muffins

2 cups whole-wheat flour
1 cup all-purpose flour
1¼ cups sugar
1 tablespoon baking powder
1 teaspoon salt

1½ cups soy milk
½ cup applesauce
½ teaspoon vanilla
2 cups blueberries, divided

1. Preheat oven to 400°F.
2. In a large bowl, combine the flours, sugar, baking powder, and salt. Set aside.
3. In a separate small bowl, whisk together the soy milk, applesauce, and vanilla until well mixed.
4. Combine the wet ingredients with the dry ingredients, stirring just until mixed. Gently fold in half of the blueberries.
5. Spoon batter into lined or greased muffin tins, filling each tin about ⅔ full. Sprinkle remaining blueberries on top of muffins.
6. Bake for 20–25 minutes or until lightly golden brown on top.

PER 1 MUFFIN	Fat: 1 g	Sodium: 201 mg	Carbohydrates: 34 g
Calories: 149	Protein: 3 g	Fiber: 2 g	Sugar: 17 g

"Chicken" Noodle Soup

If you're sick in bed, this brothy soup is just as comforting and nutritious as the real thing.

Serves 6

6 cups vegetable broth
1 medium carrot, diced
2 ribs celery, diced
1 medium onion, chopped

½ cup TVP
2 bay leaves
1½ teaspoons Italian seasoning
1 cup small pasta

Combine all ingredients in a large soup or stock pot. Cover and simmer for 15–20 minutes.

PER SERVING			
Calories: 119	Fat: 1 g Protein: 7 g	Sodium: 674 mg Fiber: 3 g	Carbohydrates: 21 g Sugar: 4 g

Super "Meaty" Chili with TVP

Any mock meat will work well in a vegetarian chili, but TVP is easy to keep on hand and very inexpensive. This is more of a thick, "meaty" Texas chili than a vegetable chili, but chili is easy and forgiving, so if you want to toss in some zucchini, broccoli, or diced carrots, by all means, do!

Serves 6

1 cup heated vegetable broth
1 tablespoon soy sauce
1½ cups TVP granules
1 medium yellow onion, chopped
5 cloves garlic, minced
2 tablespoons olive oil
1 cup corn kernels (fresh, frozen, or canned)

1 medium bell pepper, any color, chopped
2 (15-ounce) cans kidney beans, undrained
1 (15-ounce) can diced tomatoes, undrained
½ teaspoon cayenne pepper
1 teaspoon cumin
2 tablespoons chili powder

1. In a medium-sized microwave-safe bowl, combine vegetable broth and soy sauce and microwave on high for 3 minutes.
2. Place the TVP in a medium-sized heat-safe bowl. Carefully cover the TVP with the heated vegetable broth and soy sauce. Allow to sit for 3–4 minutes only, then drain.
3. In a large soup or stock pot, sauté the onion and garlic in olive oil over medium heat until onions are soft, about 3–4 minutes.
4. Add remaining ingredients and TVP, stirring well to combine. Cover and allow to simmer over low heat for at least 30 minutes, stirring occasionally.

| PER SERVING | Fat: 7 g | Sodium: 819 mg | Carbohydrates: 53 g |
| Calories: 368 | Protein: 27 g | Fiber: 15 g | Sugar: 14 g |

White Bean and Orzo Minestrone

Italian minestrone is a simple and universally loved soup. This version uses tiny orzo pasta, cannellini beans, and plenty of veggies.

Serves 6

3 cloves garlic, minced
1 medium yellow onion, peeled and chopped
2 ribs celery, chopped
2 tablespoons olive oil
5 cups vegetable broth
1 medium carrot, peeled and diced
1 cup green beans, chopped

2 small red potatoes, chopped small
2 medium tomatoes, chopped
1 (15-ounce) can cannellini beans, drained
1 teaspoon dried basil leaves
½ teaspoon oregano
¼ cup orzo
⅛ teaspoon salt
⅛ teaspoon ground black pepper

1. In a large soup pot, heat garlic, onion, and celery in olive oil until just soft, about 3–4 minutes.
2. Add vegetable broth, carrot, green beans, potatoes, tomatoes, cannellini beans, basil, and oregano and bring to a simmer. Cover and cook on medium-low heat for 20–25 minutes.
3. Add orzo and heat another 10 minutes, just until orzo is cooked. Season with salt and pepper.

PER SERVING	Fat: 6 g	Sodium: 726 mg	Carbohydrates: 35 g
Calories: 211	Protein: 7 g	Fiber: 6 g	Sugar: 7 g

Garlic Miso and Onion Soup

Boiling miso destroys some of its beneficial enzymes, so be sure to heat this soup to just below a simmer. Use a soft hand when slicing the silken tofu, so it doesn't crumble.

Serves 4

5 cups water
½ cup sliced shiitake mushrooms
3 scallions, chopped
½ medium onion, chopped
4 cloves garlic, minced

¾ teaspoon garlic powder
2 tablespoons soy sauce
1 teaspoon sesame oil
1 (16-ounce) block silken tofu, diced
⅓ cup miso

1. Combine all ingredients except for miso in a large soup or stock pot and bring to a slow simmer over medium-low heat. Cook uncovered for 10–12 minutes.
2. Reduce heat and stir in miso, being careful not to boil.
3. Heat, stirring to dissolve miso, for another 5 minutes until onions and mushrooms are soft.

PER SERVING | Fat: 6 g | Sodium: 1,368 mg | Carbohydrates: 14 g
Calories: 143 | Protein: 10 g | Fiber: 2 g | Sugar: 4 g

Cream Cheese and Butternut Squash Soup

This isn't a healthy hippie vegetable soup—it's a rich, decadent, stick-to-your-thighs soup. Nonetheless, it's absolutely delicious. Top with a mountain of homemade croutons or serve with crusty French bread.

Serves 4

2 cloves garlic, minced
½ medium yellow onion, diced
2 tablespoons olive oil
3½ cups vegetable broth
1 medium butternut squash, peeled, seeded, and chopped into cubes

1 teaspoon curry powder
¼ teaspoon nutmeg
¼ teaspoon salt
½ (8-ounce) container vegan cream cheese

1. In a large skillet or stock pot, sauté garlic and onions in olive oil over medium heat until soft, about 3–4 minutes.
2. Reduce heat to medium-low and add vegetable broth, squash, curry powder, nutmeg, and salt. Simmer for 25 minutes until squash is soft.
3. Working in batches, purée until almost smooth or to desired consistency. Or, if squash is soft enough, mash smooth with a large fork.
4. Return soup to very low heat and stir in vegan cream cheese until melted, combined, and heated through. Adjust seasonings to taste.

PER SERVING | Fat: 15 g | Sodium: 838 mg | Carbohydrates: 33 g
Calories: 264 | Protein: 15 g | Fiber: 7 g | Sugar: 8 g

Potato and Leek Soup

With simple earthy flavors, this classic soup is a comforting starter.

Serves 6

1 medium yellow onion, peeled and diced
2 cloves garlic, peeled and minced
2 tablespoons olive oil
6 cups vegetable broth
3 leeks, sliced
2 large red potatoes, chopped
2 bay leaves

1 cup unsweetened soy milk
2 tablespoons vegan margarine
¾ teaspoon salt
⅓ teaspoon black pepper
½ teaspoon dried sage
½ teaspoon dried thyme leaves
2 tablespoons nutritional yeast

1. In a large skillet or stock pot, sauté onions and garlic in olive oil over medium heat for a few minutes until onions are soft.
2. Add vegetable broth, leeks, potatoes, and bay leaves and bring to a slow simmer.
3. Allow to cook, partially covered, for 30 minutes until potatoes are soft.
4. Remove bay leaves. Working in batches as needed, purée soup in a blender until almost smooth or to desired consistency.
5. Return soup to pot and stir in remaining ingredients. Reheat as needed.

PER SERVING
Calories: 233
Fat: 9 g
Protein: 6 g
Sodium: 1,038 mg
Fiber: 5 g
Carbohydrates: 33 g
Sugar: 7 g

Vegan Mayonnaise

The secret to getting a really creamy homemade Vegan Mayonnaise is to add the oil very, very slowly—literally just a few drops at a time—and use the highest available speed on your food processor.

Makes 1 cup

1 (12-ounce) block silken tofu
1½ tablespoons lemon juice
1 teaspoon yellow mustard
1½ teaspoons apple cider vinegar

1 teaspoon sugar
¾ teaspoon onion powder
½ teaspoon salt
⅓ cup canola oil

1. Process all ingredients, except oil, in a food processor until smooth.
2. On high speed, slowly incorporate the oil just a few drops at a time until smooth and creamy.
3. Chill for at least 1 hour before serving to allow flavors to blend. Mayonnaise will also thicken as it sits.

PER 1 TABLESPOON	Fat: 3 g	Sodium: 41 mg	Carbohydrates: 1 g
Calories: 28	Protein: 1 g	Fiber: 0 g	Sugar: 0 g

Dairy-Free Ranch Dressing

An all-American creamy homemade ranch dressing, without the buttermilk. Get those baby carrots ready to dip!

Makes 1 cup

1 cup Vegan Mayonnaise (see recipe in this chapter)

¼ cup unsweetened soy milk

1 teaspoon Dijon mustard

1 tablespoon lemon juice

1 teaspoon onion powder

¾ teaspoon garlic powder

1 tablespoon minced fresh chives

1. In a large bowl, whisk or blend together all ingredients, except chives, until smooth.

2. Stir in chives until well combined.

PER 2 TABLESPOONS Fat: 4 g   Sodium: 92 mg   Carbohydrates: 2 g
Calories: 45   Protein: 1 g   Fiber: 0 g   Sugar: 1 g

Hot German Dijon Potato Salad

Tangy deli-style German potato salad requires potatoes that are thinly sliced and not over-cooked. This vegan version is just as good—if not better—than any other recipe you'll find.

Serves 4

4 large potatoes, precooked and cooled
½ medium yellow onion, sliced thin
2 tablespoons olive oil
⅓ cup water
⅓ cup white vinegar
1 tablespoon Dijon mustard

1 tablespoon whole-wheat flour
1 teaspoon granulated sugar
2 scallions, chopped
⅛ teaspoon salt
⅛ teaspoon ground black pepper

1. Slice potatoes into thin coins and set aside.
2. In a large skillet, heat onions in olive oil over medium heat and cook until just barely soft, about 2–3 minutes.
3. Reduce heat and add water, vinegar, mustard, flour, and sugar, stirring to combine. Bring to a simmer and cook until thickened, just a minute or 2.
4. Reduce heat and stir in potatoes and scallions. Season with salt and pepper.

PER SERVING	Fat: 7 g	Sodium: 232 mg	Carbohydrates: 63 g
Calories: 345	Protein: 8 g	Fiber: 7 g	Sugar: 7 g

Sesame and Soy Coleslaw Salad

You don't need mayonnaise to make a coleslaw!

Serves 4

1 medium head Napa cabbage, shredded
1 medium carrot, peeled and grated
2 green onions, chopped
1 medium red bell pepper, seeded and
  sliced thin
2 tablespoons olive oil

2 tablespoons apple cider vinegar
2 teaspoons soy sauce
½ teaspoon sesame oil
2 tablespoons maple syrup
2 tablespoons sesame seeds

1. Toss together the cabbage, carrot, green onions, and bell pepper in a large bowl.
2. In a separate small bowl, whisk together the olive oil, vinegar, soy sauce, sesame oil, and maple syrup until well combined.
3. Drizzle dressing over cabbage and veggies and toss well to combine. Top with sesame seeds and serve.

PER SERVING
Calories: 171

Fat: 10 g
Protein: 5 g

Sodium: 218 mg
Fiber: 3 g

Carbohydrates: 19 g
Sugar: 12 g

Deli-Style Macaroni Salad

A classic creamy pasta salad with Vegan Mayonnaise. Add a can of kidney beans or chickpeas for a protein boost.

Serves 6

3 cups cooked macaroni
1 medium carrot, peeled and diced small
½ cup green peas
½ cup corn
1 rib celery, diced
½ cup Vegan Mayonnaise (see recipe in this chapter)

1½ tablespoons yellow mustard
2 tablespoons apple cider vinegar
2 teaspoons sugar
2 tablespoons sweet pickle relish
2 tablespoons chopped fresh dill
⅛ teaspoon salt
⅛ teaspoon ground black pepper

1. Combine the macaroni, carrot, peas, corn, and celery in a large bowl.
2. In a separate small bowl, whisk together the mayonnaise, mustard, vinegar, sugar, and relish. Combine with macaroni.
3. Stir in the fresh dill and season with salt and pepper.
4. Chill for at least 2 hours before serving to allow flavors to combine and to soften veggies.

PER SERVING
Calories: 135

Fat: 4 g
Protein: 4 g

Sodium: 208 mg
Fiber: 3 g

Carbohydrates: 22 g
Sugar: 5 g

Kidney Bean and Chickpea Salad

This marinated two-bean salad is perfect for summer picnics or as a side for outdoor barbecues or potlucks.

Serves 6

¼ cup olive oil
¼ cup red wine vinegar
½ teaspoon paprika
2 tablespoons lemon juice
1 (14-ounce) can chickpeas, drained
1 (14-ounce) can kidney beans, drained

½ cup sliced black olives
1 (8-ounce) can corn, drained
½ red onion, chopped
1 tablespoon chopped fresh parsley
Salt and pepper to taste

1. In a medium bowl, whisk together olive oil, vinegar, paprika, and lemon juice.
2. In a large bowl, combine the chickpeas, beans, olives, corn, red onion, and parsley. Pour the olive oil dressing over the bean mixture and toss well to combine.
3. Season with salt and pepper, to taste.
4. Chill for at least 1 hour before serving to allow flavors to mingle.

PER SERVING
Calories: 226

Fat: 13 g
Protein: 7 g

Sodium: 603 mg
Fiber: 5 g

Carbohydrates: 23 g
Sugar: 5 g

Fresh Basil Bruschetta with Balsamic Reduction

Your guests will be so delighted by the rich flavors of the balsamic reduction sauce that they won't even notice that the cheese is missing from this vegan bruschetta. Use a fresh artisan bread, if you can, for extra flavor.

Serves 4

8 slices French bread
¾ cup balsamic vinegar
1 tablespoon sugar
2 large tomatoes, diced small
3 cloves garlic, minced

2 tablespoons olive oil
¼ cup chopped fresh basil
¼ teaspoon salt
⅛ teaspoon black pepper

1. Toast bread in toaster or for 5 minutes in the oven at 350°F.
2. Whisk together the balsamic vinegar and sugar in a small saucepan. Bring to a boil; then reduce to a slow simmer. Allow to cook for 6–8 minutes until almost thickened. Remove from heat.
3. Combine the tomatoes, garlic, olive oil, basil, salt, and pepper in a large bowl. Gently toss with balsamic sauce.
4. Spoon tomato and balsamic mixture over bread slices and serve immediately.

PER SERVING	Fat: 9 g	Sodium: 588 mg	Carbohydrates: 52 g
Calories: 327	Protein: 9 g	Fiber: 3 g	Sugar: 16 g

Hot Artichoke Spinach Dip

Serve this creamy dip hot with some baguette slices, crackers, pita bread, or sliced bell peppers and jicama. If you want to get fancy, you can carve out a bread bowl for an edible serving dish.

Serves 8

1 (12-ounce) package frozen spinach, thawed
1 (14-ounce) can artichoke hearts, drained
¼ cup vegan margarine, such as Earth Balance
¼ cup flour

2 cups plain unsweetened almond milk
½ cup nutritional yeast
1 teaspoon garlic powder
1½ teaspoons onion powder
¼ teaspoon salt

1. Preheat oven to 350°F. Purée spinach and artichokes in a blender until almost smooth and set aside.
2. In a small saucepan, melt the vegan margarine over low heat. Slowly whisk in flour, 1 tablespoon at a time, stirring constantly to avoid lumps, until thick.
3. Remove from heat and add spinach and artichoke mixture, stirring to combine. Add remaining ingredients.
4. Transfer to a large oven-proof casserole dish or bowl and bake for 20 minutes. Serve hot.

PER SERVING	Fat: 7 g	Sodium: 305 mg	Carbohydrates: 9 g
Calories: 114	Protein: 5 g	Fiber: 3 g	Sugar: 1 g

Fried Zucchini Sticks

You don't have to deep-fry these zucchini sticks, just sauté them in a bit of oil if you prefer. This is a great appetizer or snack for kids!

Serves 4

¾ cup flour
½ teaspoon garlic powder
¾ teaspoon Italian seasoning

¼ teaspoon salt
4 medium zucchini, cut into strips
Oil for frying

1. In a large bowl or pan, combine the flour, garlic powder, Italian seasoning, and salt.
2. Lightly toss the zucchini strips with the flour mixture, coating well.
3. Heat oil in a large skillet or frying pan over medium heat. When oil is hot, gently add zucchini strips to pan.
4. Fry until lightly golden brown on all sides. Serve with vegan ranch dressing or ketchup.

PER SERVING	Fat: 12 g	Sodium: 162 mg	Carbohydrates: 24 g
Calories: 222	Protein: 5 g	Fiber: 2 g	Sugar: 4 g

Avocado and Shiitake Pot Stickers

Once you try these California-fusion pot stickers, you'll wish you had made a double batch! These little dumplings don't need to be enhanced with a complex dipping sauce, so serve them plain or with soy sauce.

Makes 12 pot stickers

1 medium avocado, peeled, pitted, and diced small
½ cup shiitake mushrooms, diced
½ (12-ounce) block silken tofu, crumbled
1 clove garlic, minced

2 teaspoons balsamic vinegar
1 teaspoon soy sauce
12 vegan dumpling wrappers
Water for steaming

1. In a small bowl, gently mash together all ingredients, except wrappers, just until mixed and crumbly.
2. Place about 1½ teaspoons of the filling in the middle of each wrapper. Fold in half and pinch closed, forming little pleats. You may want to dip your fingertips in water to help the dumplings stay sealed if needed.
3. To steam: Carefully place a layer of dumplings in a steamer, being sure the dumplings don't touch. Place steamer above boiling water and allow to cook, covered, for 3–4 minutes.

PER 2 POT STICKERS | Fat: 6 g | Sodium: 152 mg | Carbohydrates: 14 g
Calories: 120 | Protein: 4 g | Fiber: 3 g | Sugar: 1 g

Walnut Asparagus "Egg" Rolls

It's not traditional, but it's certainly delicious. Spring roll wrappers or wonton wrappers are just fine if you can't find eggless egg roll wraps.

Makes 15 egg rolls

1 medium bunch asparagus
2 medium avocados, pitted and peeled
½ medium onion, minced
1 teaspoon lime juice
1 tablespoon soy sauce

1 teaspoon chipotle powder
½ cup walnuts, finely chopped
¼ cup chopped fresh cilantro
15 vegan egg roll wrappers
Oil for frying

1. Place the asparagus in a steamer basket over boiling water and cook until crisp-tender, then chop into ½" slices.
2. Mash together the asparagus with the avocados, onion, lime juice, soy sauce, chipotle, walnuts, and cilantro.
3. Place 2–3 tablespoons of filling in each wrapper. Fold the bottom up, then fold the sides in, and roll, wetting the edges with water to help it stick together.
4. In a large skillet, fry in hot oil for 1–2 minutes on each side.

PER 1 EGG ROLL	Fat: 12 g	Sodium: 258 mg	Carbohydrates: 23 g
Calories: 216	Protein: 5 g	Fiber: 3 g	Sugar: 1 g

Parsley and Onion Dip

If you like packaged onion dip mixes, try this tofu-based version with fresh parsley and chives. Perfect for carrots or crackers.

Serves 6

1 medium yellow onion, peeled and chopped

3 cloves garlic, peeled and minced

1 tablespoon olive oil

1 (16-ounce) block firm tofu, well pressed

½ teaspoon onion powder

3 teaspoons lemon juice

¼ cup chopped fresh parsley

2 tablespoons chopped fresh chives

¼ teaspoon salt

1. In a large skillet, sauté onions and garlic in oil for 3–4 minutes over medium heat until onions are soft. Remove from heat and allow to cool slightly.
2. Process the onion and garlic with the tofu, onion powder, and lemon juice in a food processor or blender until onion is minced and tofu is almost smooth.
3. Mash together with remaining ingredients by hand.

PER SERVING

Calories: 96

Fat: 6 g
Protein: 7 g

Sodium: 103 mg
Fiber: 1 g

Carbohydrates: 4 g
Sugar: 1 g

Nacho "Cheese" Dip

Peanut butter in cheese sauce? No, that's not a typo! Just a touch of peanut butter creates a creamy and nutty layer of flavor to this sauce and helps it to thicken nicely. Use this sauce to dress plain steamed veggies or make homemade nachos.

Makes 1 cup

3 tablespoons vegan margarine
1 cup unsweetened soy milk
¾ teaspoon garlic powder
½ teaspoon salt
½ teaspoon onion powder

1 tablespoon peanut butter
¼ cup flour
¼ cup nutritional yeast
¾ cup salsa

1. Heat margarine and soy milk together in a medium pan over low heat. Add garlic powder, salt, and onion powder, stirring to combine. Add peanut butter and stir until melted.
2. Whisk in flour, 1 tablespoon at a time, until smooth. Heat until thickened, about 5–6 minutes.
3. Stir in nutritional yeast and salsa.
4. Allow to cool slightly before serving, as cheese sauce will thicken as it cools.

PER ¼ CUP			
Calories: 199	Fat: 12 g	Sodium: 498 mg	Carbohydrates: 18 g
	Protein: 6 g	Fiber: 3 g	Sugar: 7 g

Black Bean Guacamole

Sneaking some extra fiber and protein into a traditional Mexican guacamole makes this dip a more nutritious appetizer.

Makes 2 cups

1 (15-ounce) can black beans, partially drained
3 medium avocados, pitted and peeled
1 tablespoon lime juice
½ medium red onion, peeled and diced

1 large tomato, diced
2 cloves garlic, minced
½ teaspoon chili powder
¼ teaspoon salt
1 tablespoon chopped fresh cilantro

1. Using a fork or a potato masher, mash the beans in a medium-sized bowl just until they are halfway mashed, leaving some texture.
2. Combine all the remaining ingredients and mash together until mixed.
3. Allow to sit for at least 10 minutes before serving to allow the flavors to set.
4. Gently mix again just before serving.

PER ¼ CUP			
Calories: 66	Fat: 4 g	Sodium: 58 mg	Carbohydrates: 6 g
	Protein: 2 g	Fiber: 4 g	Sugar: 0 g

Mango Citrus Salsa

Salsa has a variety of uses, and this recipe adds color and variety to your usual chips and dip or Mexican dishes.

Makes 2 cups

1 medium mango, peeled and chopped

2 medium tangerines, peeled and chopped

½ medium red bell pepper, peeled and chopped

½ medium red onion, peeled and minced

3 cloves garlic, minced

½ medium jalapeño pepper, seeded and minced

2 tablespoons lime juice

½ teaspoon salt

¼ teaspoon black pepper

3 tablespoons chopped fresh cilantro

1. Gently toss together all ingredients in a medium bowl.
2. Allow to sit for at least 15 minutes before serving to allow flavors to mingle.

PER ¼ CUP
Calories: 32

Fat: 0 g
Protein: 0 g

Sodium: 104 mg
Fiber: 2 g

Carbohydrates: 8 g
Sugar: 6 g

Creamed Spinach and Mushrooms

The combination of greens and nutritional yeast is simply delicious and provides an excellent jolt of nutrients that vegans need. Don't forget that spinach will shrink when cooked, so use lots!

Serves 4

½ medium onion, diced

2 cloves garlic, minced

1½ cups sliced mushrooms

2 tablespoons olive oil

1 tablespoon flour

2 large bunches fresh spinach, trimmed

1 cup soy milk

1 tablespoon vegan margarine

¼ teaspoon nutmeg

2 tablespoons nutritional yeast

¼ teaspoon salt

⅛ teaspoon black pepper

1. In a large skillet, sauté onion, garlic, and mushrooms in olive oil for 3–4 minutes over medium heat. Add flour and heat, stirring constantly, for 1 minute.
2. Reduce heat to medium-low and add spinach and soy milk. Cook uncovered for 8–10 minutes until spinach is soft and liquid has reduced.
3. Stir in remaining ingredients and season with salt and pepper.

PER SERVING

Calories: 177

Fat: 11 g

Protein: 8 g

Sodium: 304 mg

Fiber: 4 g

Carbohydrates: 14 g

Sugar: 4 g

Cajun Collard Greens

Like Brussels sprouts and kimchi, collard greens are one of those foods folks tend to either love or hate. They're highly nutritious, so hopefully this recipe will turn you into a lover, if you're not already.

Serves 4

1 medium onion, diced
3 cloves garlic, minced
1 pound collard greens, chopped
2 tablespoons olive oil
¾ cup water or vegetable broth

1 (14-ounce) can diced tomatoes, drained
1½ teaspoons Cajun seasoning
½ teaspoon hot sauce
¼ teaspoon salt

1. In a large skillet, sauté onions, garlic, and collard greens in olive oil for 3–5 minutes over medium heat until onions are soft.
2. Add water or vegetable broth, tomatoes, and Cajun seasoning. Bring to a simmer, cover, and allow to cook for 20 minutes or until greens are soft, stirring occasionally.
3. Remove lid, stir in hot sauce and salt, and cook uncovered for another minute or 2, to allow excess moisture to evaporate.

PER SERVING	Fat: 8 g	Sodium: 478 mg	Carbohydrates: 18 g
Calories: 151	Protein: 6 g	Fiber: 8 g	Sugar: 6 g

Potatoes "Au Gratin" Casserole

You'll never miss the boxed version after trying these easy potatoes!

Serves 4

4 large potatoes
1 medium onion, chopped
1 tablespoon vegan margarine
2 tablespoons flour
2 cups unsweetened soy milk
2 teaspoons onion powder

1 teaspoon garlic powder
2 tablespoons nutritional yeast
1 teaspoon lemon juice
½ teaspoon salt
¾ teaspoon paprika
½ teaspoon black pepper

1. Preheat oven to 375°F.
2. Slice potatoes into thin coins and arrange half the slices in a large casserole or baking dish. Layer half of the onions on top of the potatoes.
3. In a large saucepan, melt the margarine over low heat and add flour, stirring to make a paste. Add soy milk, onion powder, garlic powder, nutritional yeast, lemon juice, and salt, stirring to combine. Stir over low heat until sauce has thickened, about 2–3 minutes.
4. Pour half of sauce over potatoes and onions, then layer the remaining potatoes and onions on top of the sauce. Pour the remaining sauce on top.
5. Sprinkle with paprika and black pepper and top with bread crumbs or French-fried onions.
6. Cover and bake for 45 minutes and then an additional 10 minutes uncovered.

PER SERVING

Calories: 279	Fat: 5 g / Protein: 10 g	Sodium: 423 mg / Fiber: 7 g	Carbohydrates: 49 g / Sugar: 9 g

Roasted Brussels Sprouts with Apples

Brussels sprouts are surprisingly delicious when prepared properly, so if you have bad memories of being force-fed soggy, limp baby cabbages as a child, don't let that stop you from trying this recipe!

Serves 4

2 cups Brussels sprouts, chopped into quarters
8 whole cloves garlic, peeled
2 tablespoons olive oil

2 tablespoons balsamic vinegar
¾ teaspoon salt
½ teaspoon black pepper
2 medium apples, cored and chopped

1. Preheat oven to 425°F.
2. Arrange Brussels sprouts and garlic in a single layer on a baking sheet. Drizzle with olive oil and balsamic vinegar and season with salt and pepper. Roast for 10–12 minutes, tossing once.
3. Remove tray from oven and add apples, tossing gently to combine. Roast for 10 more minutes or until apples are soft, tossing once again.

PER SERVING	Fat: 7 g	Sodium: 451 mg	Carbohydrates: 20 g
Calories: 143	Protein: 2 g	Fiber: 4 g	Sugar: 12 g

Gingered and Pralined Sweet Potatoes

Keep this recipe handy during the holiday season. Who needs marshmallows anyway?

Serves 4

4 large sweet potatoes, peeled and baked
¼ cup soy cream
¼ cup no-pulp orange juice
½ teaspoon salt
½ cup chopped pecans

2 tablespoons vegan margarine
⅓ cup maple syrup
⅓ cup flour
½ cup candied ginger

1. Preheat oven to 350°F.
2. In a large bowl, mash together the sweet potatoes, soy cream or soy milk, orange juice, and salt until smooth and creamy. Transfer to a lightly greased large casserole dish.
3. In a small bowl, combine the remaining ingredients and spread over the top of the sweet potatoes.
4. Bake for 30 minutes.

PER SERVING
Calories: 456

Fat: 18 g
Protein: 5 g

Sodium: 406 mg
Fiber: 6 g

Carbohydrates: 71 g
Sugar: 40 g

Classic Green Bean Casserole

Shop for a vegan cream of mushroom soup to use in your traditional holiday recipe or try this easy homemade vegan version. Delish!

Serves 4

1 (12-ounce) bag frozen green beans
¾ cup sliced mushrooms
2 tablespoons vegan margarine
2 tablespoons flour
1½ cups unsweetened soy milk
1 tablespoon Dijon mustard

½ teaspoon garlic powder
½ teaspoon salt
¼ teaspoon sage
¼ teaspoon oregano
¼ teaspoon black pepper
1½ cups French-fried onions

1. Preheat oven to 375°F. Place green beans and mushrooms in a large casserole dish.
2. In a medium-sized saucepan, melt vegan margarine over low heat. Stir in flour until pasty and combined. Add soy milk, mustard, garlic powder, salt, sage, oregano, and pepper, stirring continuously to combine until thickened.
3. Pour sauce over mushrooms and green beans and top with French-fried onions.
4. Bake for 16–18 minutes until onions are lightly browned and toasted.

PER SERVING	Fat: 18 g	Sodium: 669 mg	Carbohydrates: 23 g
Calories: 274	Protein: 5 g	Fiber: 3 g	Sugar: 5 g

Caramelized Onion and Barbecue Sauce Pizza

Cheeseless pizza is more delicious than you might think. Sprinkle it with nutritional yeast if you want that cheesy flavor or make some Dairy-Free Ranch Dressing (see recipe in this chapter) to dip it in.

Serves 4

⅔ cup barbecue sauce
1 (9") vegan pizza crust or pizza dough
2 medium red onions, peeled and chopped
3 tablespoons olive oil
1 (16-ounce) block tofu, diced small

½ cup diced canned pineapple, drained
⅓ teaspoon garlic powder
⅛ teaspoon salt
⅛ teaspoon black pepper

1. Preheat oven to 450°F. Spread barbecue sauce on pizza crust.
2. In a medium sauté pan, heat onions in olive oil for 2–3 minutes, stirring occasionally. Add tofu and sauté until tofu is lightly crisped and onions are soft and caramelized.
3. Top pizza with tofu, onions, and pineapple. Sprinkle with garlic powder and salt and pepper.
4. Place pizza directly on oven rack and bake for 12–14 minutes or according to instructions on pizza dough. Pizza is done when bottom of crust is lightly browned.

PER SERVING			
Calories: 448	Fat: 18 g	Sodium: 984 mg	Carbohydrates: 55 g
	Protein: 16 g	Fiber: 4 g	Sugar: 21 g

Breaded Eggplant "Parmesan"

Slowly baking these breaded eggplant cutlets brings out the best flavor, but they can also be panfried in a bit of oil.

Serves 4

1 medium eggplant
½ teaspoon salt
¾ cup flour
1 teaspoon garlic powder
⅔ cup unsweetened soy milk
Egg replacer for 2 eggs

1½ cups bread crumbs
2 tablespoons Italian seasoning
¼ cup nutritional yeast
1½ cups marinara sauce
1 (8-ounce) package shredded mozzarella-
    flavored vegan cheese

1. Preheat oven to 400°F. Slice eggplant into ¾"-thick slices and sprinkle with salt. Allow to sit for 10 minutes. Gently pat dry to remove extra moisture.
2. In a shallow bowl or pie tin, combine flour and garlic powder. In a separate small bowl, whisk together the soy milk and egg replacer. In a third small bowl, combine the bread crumbs, Italian seasoning, and nutritional yeast.
3. Coat each eggplant slice with the flour mixture, then carefully dip in the soy milk mixture, then coat with the bread crumb mixture and place in a lightly greased large casserole dish.
4. Bake for 20–25 minutes. Remove from the oven, cover in marinara sauce, and sprinkle on cheese, then bake for another 5 minutes.

PER SERVING			
Calories: 476	Fat: 18 g	Sodium: 1,458 mg	Carbohydrates: 68 g
	Protein: 13 g	Fiber: 13 g	Sugar: 14 g

The Easiest Black Bean Burger Recipe in the World

Veggie burgers are notorious for falling apart. If you're sick of crumbly burgers, try this simple method for making black bean patties. It's 100 percent guaranteed to stick together.

Makes 6 patties

1 (15-ounce) can black beans, drained
3 tablespoons minced onions
1 teaspoon salt
1½ teaspoons garlic powder

2 teaspoons chopped parsley
1 teaspoon chili powder
⅔ cup flour
Oil for panfrying

1. Process the black beans in a blender or food processor until halfway mashed, or mash with a fork.
2. Add minced onions, salt, garlic powder, parsley, and chili powder and mash to combine.
3. Add flour, a bit at time, again mashing together to combine. You may need a little bit more or less than ⅔ cup. Beans should stick together completely.
4. Form into six patties and panfry in a medium skillet over medium heat in a bit of oil for 2–3 minutes on each side. Patties will appear to be done on the outside while still a bit mushy on the inside, so fry them a few minutes longer than you think they need.

PER 1 PATTY	Fat: 6 g	Sodium: 519 mg	Carbohydrates: 21 g
Calories: 156	Protein: 6 g	Fiber: 6 g	Sugar: 1 g

Savory Stuffed Acorn Squash

All the flavors of fall baked into one nutritious dish. Use fresh herbs if you have them and breathe deep to savor the impossibly magical aromas coming from your kitchen.

Serves 4

2 medium acorn squash
1 teaspoon garlic powder
½ teaspoon salt
2 ribs celery, chopped
1 medium onion, diced
½ cup sliced mushrooms
2 tablespoons vegan margarine
¼ cup chopped walnuts

1 tablespoon soy sauce
1 teaspoon parsley
½ teaspoon thyme
½ teaspoon sage
½ teaspoon salt
¼ teaspoon pepper
½ cup grated vegan cheese

1. Preheat oven to 350°F. Chop the squash in half lengthwise and scrape out any stringy bits and seeds.
2. Sprinkle squash with garlic powder and salt, then place cut-side down on a baking sheet and bake for 30 minutes or until almost soft; remove from oven.
3. In a large skillet, heat celery, onion, and mushrooms in vegan margarine over medium heat until soft, about 4–5 minutes.
4. Add walnuts, soy sauce, parsley, thyme, and sage, stirring to combine well, and season with salt and pepper. Heat for another minute or 2 until fragrant.
5. Fill squash with mushroom mixture and sprinkle with vegan cheese. Bake another 5–10 minutes until squash is soft.

PER SERVING	Fat: 17 g	Sodium: 1,188 mg	Carbohydrates: 34 g
Calories: 286	Protein: 4 g	Fiber: 5 g	Sugar: 7 g

Chickpea Soft Tacos

For an easy and healthy taco filling wrapped up in flour tortillas, try using chickpeas! Short on time? Pick up taco seasoning packets to use instead of the spice blend—but watch out for added MSG. You can top these tacos with fresh cilantro, shredded lettuce, black olives, vegan cheese, and nondairy sour cream.

Serves 6

2 (15-ounce) cans chickpeas, drained
½ cup water
1 (6-ounce) can tomato paste
1 tablespoon chili powder

1 teaspoon garlic powder
½ teaspoon onion powder
½ teaspoon cumin
6 (8") flour tortillas

1. Combine chickpeas, water, tomato paste, chili powder, garlic powder, onion powder, and cumin in a large skillet. Cover and simmer for 10 minutes over medium-low heat, stirring occasionally. Uncover and simmer another minute or 2 until most of the liquid is absorbed.
2. Use a fork or potato masher to mash the chickpea mixture until half mashed.
3. Spoon mixture into flour tortillas, add desired toppings, and wrap.

PER SERVING
Calories: 250

Fat: 5 g
Protein: 9 g

Sodium: 398 mg
Fiber: 6 g

Carbohydrates: 44 g
Sugar: 5 g

Cheesy Macaroni and "Hamburger" Casserole

Reminiscent of the boxed version, this is guilt-free vegan comfort food at its finest.

Serves 6

1 (12-ounce) bag macaroni noodles
4 veggie burgers, thawed and crumbled
1 medium tomato, diced
1 tablespoon olive oil
1 teaspoon chili powder
1 cup soy milk
2 tablespoons vegan margarine

2 tablespoons flour
1 teaspoon garlic powder
1 teaspoon onion powder
¼ cup nutritional yeast
¼ teaspoon salt
⅛ teaspoon black pepper

1. Prepare macaroni noodles according to package instructions.
2. In a medium pan, sauté the veggie burgers and tomatoes in oil until burgers are lightly browned, then season with chili powder.
3. In a separate small skillet, melt together the soy milk and margarine over low heat until well mixed. Stir in flour and heat until thickened, then stir in garlic powder, onion powder, and nutritional yeast and remove from heat.
4. Combine macaroni, veggie burgers, tomatoes, and sauce, gently tossing to coat.
5. Season with salt and pepper and allow to cool slightly before serving to allow ingredients to combine.

PER SERVING	Fat: 10 g	Sodium: 623 mg	Carbohydrates: 61 g
Calories: 377	Protein: 13 g	Fiber: 7 g	Sugar: 4 g

Strawberry Coconut Ice Cream

Rich and creamy, this is the most decadent dairy-free strawberry ice cream you'll ever taste.

Serves 6

2 cups coconut cream
1¾ cups frozen strawberries
¾ cup sugar

2 teaspoons vanilla
¼ teaspoon salt

1. Purée together all ingredients in a blender until smooth and creamy.
2. Transfer mixture to a large freezer-proof baking or casserole dish and freeze.
3. Stir every 30 minutes until a smooth ice cream forms, about 4 hours. If mixture gets too firm, transfer to a blender, process until smooth, then return to freezer.

PER SERVING
Calories: 479

Fat: 17 g
Protein: 1 g

Sodium: 135 mg
Fiber: 1 g

Carbohydrates: 83 g
Sugar: 79 g

Maple Date Carrot Cake

Free of refined sugar and with applesauce for moisture and just a touch of oil, this is a cake you can feel good about eating for breakfast. Leave out the dates if you want even less natural sugar.

Serves 8

1½ cups raisins
1⅓ cups pineapple juice
6 dates, diced
2¼ cups grated carrots
½ cup maple syrup
¼ cup applesauce
2 tablespoons oil

3 cups flour
1½ teaspoons baking soda
½ teaspoon salt
1 teaspoon cinnamon
½ teaspoon allspice or nutmeg
Egg replacer for 2 eggs

1. Preheat oven to 375°F and grease and flour a 9" round cake pan.
2. Combine the raisins with pineapple juice and allow to sit for 5–10 minutes to soften. In a separate small bowl, cover the dates with water until soft, about 10 minutes. Drain water from dates.
3. In a large mixing bowl, combine the raisins and pineapple juice, dates, carrots, maple syrup, applesauce, and oil. In a separate large bowl, combine the flour, baking soda, salt, cinnamon, and allspice or nutmeg.
4. Combine the dry ingredients with the wet ingredients and add egg replacer. Mix well.
5. Pour batter into prepared cake pan and bake for 30 minutes or until a toothpick inserted in the center comes out clean.

PER SERVING

Calories: 385	Fat: 5 g	Sodium: 242 mg	Carbohydrates: 87 g
	Protein: 6 g	Fiber: 8 g	Sugar: 51 g

Foolproof Vegan Fudge

Vegan fudge is much easier to make than nonvegan fudge, so don't worry about a thing when making this fudge. Regular soy milk will work just fine, but the soy cream has a richer taste.

Makes 24 (1") pieces

½ cup vegan margarine
⅓ cup cocoa
⅓ cup soy cream
½ teaspoon vanilla extract

2 tablespoons peanut butter
3½ cups powdered sugar
¾ cup finely chopped walnuts

1. Lightly grease a small baking dish or square cake pan.
2. Using a double broiler, or over very low heat in a small saucepan, melt the vegan margarine with the cocoa, soy cream, vanilla, and peanut butter.
3. Slowly incorporate powdered sugar until mixture is smooth, creamy, and thick. Stir in nuts.
4. Immediately transfer to pan and chill until completely firm, at least 2 hours.

PER 1" PIECE	Fat: 7 g	Sodium: 43 mg	Carbohydrates: 19 g
Calories: 142	Protein: 1 g	Fiber: 1 g	Sugar: 17 g

Classic Chocolate Chip Cookies

Just like Mom used to make, only with a bit of applesauce to cut down on the fat.

Makes 24 cookies

⅔ cup vegan margarine
⅔ cup granulated sugar
⅔ cup light brown sugar
⅓ cup unsweetened applesauce
1½ teaspoons vanilla
Egg replacer for 2 eggs

2½ cups flour
1 teaspoon baking soda
½ teaspoon baking powder
1 teaspoon salt
⅔ cup quick-cooking oats
1½ cups vegan chocolate chips

1. Preheat oven to 375°F.
2. In a large mixing bowl, cream together the vegan margarine and white sugar, then mix in brown sugar, applesauce, vanilla, and egg replacer.
3. In a separate large bowl, combine the flour, baking soda, baking powder, and salt, then combine with the wet ingredients. Mix well.
4. Stir in oats and chocolate chips just until combined.
5. Drop by generous spoonfuls onto a prepared baking sheet and bake for 10–12 minutes. For a chewy cookie, don't be tempted to overbake them!

PER 1 COOKIE	Fat: 9 g	Sodium: 213 mg	Carbohydrates: 28 g
Calories: 186	Protein: 2 g	Fiber: 2 g	Sugar: 18 g

Apricot Ginger Sorbet

Made with real fruit and without dairy, this is a nearly fat-free treat that you can add to smoothies or just enjoy outside on a hot summer day.

Serves 6

⅔ cup water
⅔ cup sugar
2 teaspoons fresh minced ginger

5 cups chopped apricots, fresh or frozen
3 tablespoons lemon juice

1. In a medium pan, bring the water, sugar, and ginger to a boil, then reduce to a slow simmer. Heat for 3–4 more minutes until sugar is dissolved and a syrup forms. Allow to cool.
2. In a blender, purée the sugar syrup, apricots, and lemon juice until smooth.
3. Transfer mixture to a large freezer-proof baking or casserole dish and freeze.
4. Stir every 30 minutes until a smooth ice cream forms, about 4 hours. If mixture gets too firm, transfer to a blender, process until smooth, then return to freezer.

PER SERVING
Calories: 157

Fat: 1 g
Protein: 2 g

Sodium: 2 mg
Fiber: 3 g

Carbohydrates: 39 g
Sugar: 35 g

Sweetheart Raspberry Lemon Cupcakes

Add half a teaspoon of lemon extract for extra lemony goodness to these sweet and tart cupcakes. Or omit the raspberries and add 3 tablespoons of poppy seeds for lemon poppy seed cupcakes. Sweet and tart—sweetheart! Get it?

Makes 18 cupcakes

½ cup vegan margarine, softened
1 cup sugar
½ teaspoon vanilla
¾ cup vanilla soy milk
2 tablespoons lemon juice
Zest from 2 lemons

1¾ cups flour
1½ teaspoons baking powder
½ teaspoon baking soda
¼ teaspoon salt
¾ cup diced raspberries, fresh or frozen

1. Preheat oven to 350°F and grease or line a cupcake tin.
2. In a small bowl, beat together the margarine and sugar until light and fluffy, then add vanilla, soy milk, lemon juice, and zest.
3. In a separate small bowl, sift together the flour, baking powder, baking soda, and salt.
4. Combine flour mixture with wet ingredients just until mixed. Do not overmix. Gently fold in diced raspberries.
5. Fill cupcake tins about ⅔ full with batter and bake immediately for 16–18 minutes or until done.

PER 1 CUPCAKE
Calories: 126
Fat: 5 g
Protein: 1 g
Sodium: 155 mg
Fiber: 1 g
Carbohydrates: 19 g
Sugar: 12 g

Chocolate Graham Cracker Candy Bars

Have the kids help out by spreading the peanut butter while you do the dipping. Matzo, saltines, or any cracker will work, really, and because half of them will disappear before you're finished making them, you may want to make a double—or even triple—batch!

Makes 16 bars

1 cup almond butter
8 vegan graham crackers, broken into
   quarters
1 cup vegan chocolate chips

¼ cup vegan margarine
½ cup coconut flakes
¼ cup chopped raw walnuts

1. Line a baking pan with wax paper.
2. Spread 1 tablespoon almond butter on each cracker, then top with another cracker to make a "sandwich."
3. In a double boiler or small saucepan over very low heat, melt together the chocolate chips and margarine until smooth and creamy.
4. Using tongs, dip each cracker sandwich into melted chips to cover. Set the sandwiches back on the baking sheet and sprinkle with coconut and walnuts.
5. Chill until firm, about 1 hour.

PER 1 BAR
Calories: 211

Fat: 17 g
Protein: 4 g

Sodium: 83 mg
Fiber: 3 g

Carbohydrates: 13 g
Sugar: 8 g

Tropical Cashew Nut Butter

You can make a homemade cashew nut butter with any kind of oil, so feel free to substitute using whatever you have on hand, but you're in for a real treat when you use coconut oil in this recipe!

Makes ¾ cup

2 cups roasted cashews
½ teaspoon sugar

¼ teaspoon salt
4 tablespoons coconut oil

1. Process the cashews, sugar, and salt in a food processor on high speed until finely ground. Continue processing until cashews form a thick paste.
2. Slowly add coconut oil until smooth and creamy, scraping down sides and adding a little more oil as needed.

PER 2 TABLESPOONS	Fat: 16 g	Sodium: 56 mg	Carbohydrates: 8 g
Calories: 187	Protein: 4 g	Fiber: 1 g	Sugar: 1 g

Vegan Chocolate Hazelnut Spread

Treat yourself or your family with this rich, sticky chocolate spread. This one will have you dancing around the kitchen and licking your spoons!

Makes 1 cup

2 cups hazelnuts, chopped
½ cup cocoa powder
¾ cup powdered sugar

½ teaspoon vanilla
4 tablespoons vegetable oil

1. Process hazelnuts in a food processor until very finely ground, about 3–4 minutes.
2. Add cocoa powder, sugar, and vanilla, and process to combine.
3. Add oil, just a little bit at a time, until mixture is soft and creamy and desired consistency is reached. You may need to add a bit more or less than 4 tablespoons.

PER 2 TABLESPOONS Fat: 15 g   Sodium: 1 mg   Carbohydrates: 10 g
Calories: 174   Protein: 3 g   Fiber: 3 g   Sugar: 6 g

Carob Peanut Butter Banana Smoothie

Yummy enough for a dessert but healthy enough for breakfast, this smoothie is also a great protein boost after a sweaty workout at the gym. Use cocoa powder if you don't have any carob.

Serves 2

7–8 ice cubes
2 bananas
2 tablespoons peanut butter

2 tablespoons carob powder
1 cup soy milk

Blend together all ingredients until smooth.

PER SERVING			
Calories: 280	Fat: 11 g	Sodium: 69 mg	Carbohydrates: 44 g
	Protein: 9 g	Fiber: 8 g	Sugar: 24 g

Strawberry Protein Smoothie

Add silken tofu to a simple fruit smoothie for a creamy protein boost.

Serves 2

½ cup frozen strawberries
½ (16-ounce) block silken tofu
1 medium banana, peeled

¾ cup apple juice
4 ice cubes
1 tablespoon agave nectar

Blend together all ingredients until smooth and creamy.

PER SERVING			
Calories: 184	Fat: 3 g	Sodium: 10 mg	Carbohydrates: 37 g
	Protein: 5 g	Fiber: 3 g	Sugar: 27 g

Chai Tea

Store any leftover tea in a covered container in the refrigerator. It can be reheated, but leftover tea is best served over ice.

Serves 12

5 cups water
6 slices fresh ginger
1 teaspoon whole cloves
2 (3") cinnamon sticks
1½ teaspoons freshly ground nutmeg

½ teaspoon ground cardamom
1 cup maple syrup
12 bags black tea
6 cups coconut milk

1. Pour water into a 4-quart slow cooker. Put ginger and cloves in a muslin spice bag or a piece of cheesecloth secured with kitchen twine; add to the cooker along with cinnamon sticks, nutmeg, and cardamom. Cover and cook on low for 4–6 hours or on high for 2–3 hours.
2. Stir in maple syrup until it's dissolved into the water. Add tea bags and coconut milk; cover and cook on low for 30 minutes. Remove and discard the spices in the muslin bag or cheesecloth, the cinnamon sticks, and the tea bags. Ladle into teacups or mugs to serve.

PER SERVING
Calories: 97

Fat: 3 g
Protein: 1 g

Sodium: 14 mg
Fiber: 0 g

Carbohydrates: 19 g
Sugar: 16 g

Avocado Smoothie

This quick blended smoothie is a sweet treat when you're looking for something refreshing that resembles a milkshake.

Serves 1

1 large ripe avocado, pitted and peeled
1 cup coconut milk
½ cup almond milk

3 tablespoons maple syrup
3–4 ice cubes

In a blender, combine all ingredients until smooth. Serve chilled.

PER SERVING
Calories: 547

Fat: 36 g
Protein: 6 g

Sodium: 129 mg
Fiber: 13 g

Carbohydrates: 59 g
Sugar: 38 g

The Green Bloody Mary

This green version of the Bloody Mary has all of the necessary ingredients to repair exactly what the alcoholic version destroys!

Serves 2

1 cup chopped watercress
2 large tomatoes
2 stalks celery
½ large lemon, peeled

1 tablespoon horseradish
½ teaspoon cayenne pepper
1 cup water, divided

1. Place watercress, tomatoes, celery, lemon, horseradish, cayenne, and ½ cup water in a blender and blend until thoroughly combined.
2. Add remaining ½ cup water while blending until desired texture is achieved.

PER SERVING
Calories: 49

Fat: 1 g
Protein: 2 g

Sodium: 80 mg
Fiber: 3 g

Carbohydrates: 10 g
Sugar: 6 g

Homemade Tomato Juice

This thirst quencher is loaded with electrolytes to help you rehydrate and replenish after working out. It's an all-natural "energy drink"!

Serves 4

10 large tomatoes, seeded and sliced
1 teaspoon lemon juice

¼ teaspoon ground black pepper
1 tablespoon maple syrup

1. Place tomatoes in a 2-quart slow cooker. Cover; cook on low for 4–6 hours.
2. Press cooked tomatoes through a sieve. Add remaining ingredients and chill.

PER SERVING
Calories: 96

Fat: 1 g
Protein: 4 g

Sodium: 23 mg
Fiber: 6 g

Carbohydrates: 21 g
Sugar: 15 g

Nutritional Information for 200+ Common Vegan Foods

Here are more than 200 common foods that you can safely include in a vegan diet. Though it never hurts to check the label of processed foods, all of the foods included here are free of animal additives. This list will come in handy at the grocery store when you're wondering what to eat. You can also use this list to plan well-balanced vegan meals. Skim the list to find a few foods you already enjoy that are high in calcium, iron, and zinc, and make a note to include these nutrient-rich foods in your diet regularly.

Beverages

Food	Serving Size	Calories	Fat	Protein	Sodium	Fiber
Carrot juice	1 cup	94	0.35 g	2.2 g	68 mg	1.9 g
Coconut water	1 cup	45	0.53 g	2.4 g	250 mg	2.4 g
Coffee	8 fl oz.	5	0 g	0 g	5.3 mg	0 g
Cranberry juice	1 cup	144	0 g	0 g	5 mg	0.3 g
Grapefruit juice	1 cup	95	0.27 g	2.4 g	2.4 mg	0 g
Lemonade	1 cup	99	0 g	0 g	7 mg	0.2 g
Orange juice	1 cup	110	0 g	2 g	0 mg	0.5 g
Prune juice	½ cup	91	0 g	0.78 g	5.1 mg	1.3 g
Tea, black	1 cup	2	0 g	0 g	0 mg	0 g
Tea, green	1 cup	3	0 g	0 g	2.7 mg	0 g
Tomato juice (no added salt)	1 cup	41	0.1 g	1.8 g	24.3 mg	1 g
Water	1 cup	0	0 g	0 g	0 mg	0 g

Dairy Replacements

Food	Serving Size	Calories	Fat	Protein	Sodium	Fiber
Apple butter	2 T.	40	0 g	0 g	0 mg	2 g
Almond milk, sweetened	1 cup	60	2.5 g	1 g	150 mg	1 g

Carbohydrates	Sugar	Zinc	Calcium	Iron	Vitamin D	Vitamin B_{12}
22 g	9.2 g	0.42 mg	57 mg	1.1 mg	0 mcg	0 mcg
9.5 g	7.1 g	0 mg	57 mg	0 mg	0 mcg	0 mcg
1.3 g	0 g	0 mg	5.3 mg	0 mg	0 mcg	0 mcg
36 g	4 g	0 mg	8 mg	0.4 mg	0 mcg	0 mcg
22 g	22 g	0 mg	22 mg	0 mg	0 mcg	0 mcg
26 g	0 g	0 mg	7 mg	0.4 mg	0 mcg	0 mcg
26 g	22 g	0 mg	27.3 mg	0.5 mg	0 mcg	0 mcg
22 g	21 g	0.27 mg	15 mg	1.5 mg	0 mcg	0 mcg
0.71 g	0 g	0.024 mg	0 mg	0.024 mg	0 mcg	0 mcg
0 g	0 g	0 mg	0 mg	0.13 mg	0 mcg	0 mcg
10.3 g	8.6 g	0.4 mg	24.3 mg	1.0 mg	0 IU	0 mcg
0 g	0 g	0 mg	0 mg	0 mg	0 mcg	0 mcg

Carbohydrates	Sugar	Zinc	Calcium	Iron	Vitamin D	Vitamin B_{12}
8 g	8 g	0 mg	1.9 mg	0 mg	0 mcg	0 mcg
8 g	7 g	1.5 mg	450 mg	0.7 mg	100 IU	3 mcg

Almond milk, unsweetened	1 cup	40	4 g	1 g	180 mg	1 g
Rice milk	1 cup	120	2 g	0.4 g	86 mg	0 g
Soy hot chocolate	1 cup	100	2 g	6 g	95 mg	1 g
Soy milk	1 cup	90	4.5 g	7 g	29 mg	2 g
Soy milk, chocolate	1 cup	120	2.5 g	5 g	140 mg	3 g
Soy yogurt	1 cup	140	2.5 g	5 g	20 mg	0.5 g
Tofu crumbles	¼ (12-ounce) block	178	12 g	15 g	2 mg	1 g
Vegan cheese	1 slice	40	2 g	1 g	120 mg	0 g
Vegan cream cheese	2 T.	90	8 g	2 g	115 mg	2 g
Vegan sour cream	2 T.	28	1.9 g	3 g	85 mg	0 g

Fruits

Food	Serving Size	Calories	Fat	Protein	Sodium	Fiber
Apple	1 small	77.5	0.3 g	0.4 g	1.5 mg	3.6 g
Apricots	1 cup, halved	74.4	0.6 g	2.2 g	1.6 mg	3.1 g
Avocado	1 oz.	44.8	4.1 g	0.6 g	2 mg	2 g
Banana	1 small	89.9	0.3 g	1.1 g	1 mg	2.6 g
Blackberries	1 cup	62	0.64 g	1.4 g	1.4 mg	7.2 g
Blueberries	1 cup	84.4	0.5 g	1.1 g	1.5 mg	3.6 g
Cantaloupe melon	1 cup, balls	60.2	0.3 g	1.5 g	28.3 mg	1.6 g
Cherries	1 cup	86.9	0.3 g	1.5 g	0 mg	2.9 g
Coconut	½ cup	136	13 g	1.2 g	7.7 mg	3.5 g
Cranberries	1 oz.	86.2	0.4 g	0 g	0.8 mg	1.6 g
Currants	1 cup	63	0.25 g	1.1 g	1.1 mg	4.5 g
Dates	1 fruit	66.5	0 g	0.4 g	0.2 mg	1.6 g
Figs	1 fruit	46	0.21 g	0.63 g	0.63 mg	1.9 g
Grapes	1 cup	61	0.3 g	0.91 g	1.8 mg	0.91 g
Grapefruit	1 large	107	0.37 g	3.3 g	0 mg	3.3 g
Honeydew melon	1 cup	64	0.2 g	1.8 g	32 mg	1.8 g
Kiwi	1 fruit	55	0.91 g	0.91 g	2.7 mg	2.7 g
Kumquats	4 fruits	54	0.75 g	1.5 g	7.5 mg	5.3 g

2 g	0 g	0 mg	450 mg	4%	0 mcg	0 mcg
24 g	0 g	0 mg	20 mg	0.2 mg	0 mcg	0 mcg
20 g	15 g	4%	300 mg	6%	30%	50%
5 g	1 g	0 mg	80 mg	1.4 mg	3 mcg	0.36 mg
19 g	16 g	0.6 mg	300 mg	1.08 mg	0 IU	3 mcg
28 g	19 g	0 mg	8 mg	0 mg	0 IU	0 mcg
5 g	0 g	2 mg	421 mg	3 mg	0 mcg	0 mcg
5 g	0 g	0 mg	200 mg	0 mg	0 IU	0 mcg
3 g	1 g	0 mg	20 mg	0.36 mg	0 IU	0 mcg
<1 g	0 g	0 mg	0 mg	0 mg	0 IU	0 mcg

Carbohydrates	Sugar	Zinc	Calcium	Iron	Vitamin D	Vitamin B_{12}
20.6 g	15.5 g	0.1 mg	8.9 mg	0.2 mg	0 IU	0 mcg
17.4 g	14.3 g	0.3 mg	20.2 mg	0.6 mg	0 mcg	0 mcg
2.4 g	0.2 g	0.2 mg	3.4 mg	0.2 mg	0 IU	0 mcg
23.1 g	12.4 g	0.2 mg	5.1 mg	0.3 mg	0 IU	0 mcg
14 g	7.2 g	1.4 mg	42 mg	1.4 mg	0 mcg	0 mcg
21.4 g	14.7 g	0.2 mg	8.9 mg	0.4 mg	0 IU	0 mcg
15.6 g	13.9 g	0.3 mg	15.9 mg	0.4 mg	0 mcg	0 mcg
22.1 g	17.7 g	0.1 mg	17.9 mg	0.5 mg	0 mcg	0 mcg
5.8 g	2.3 g	0.38 mg	5.4 mg	0.77 mg	0 mcg	0 mcg
23.1 g	18.2 g	0 mg	2.8 mg	0.1 mg	0 mcg	0 mcg
16 g	7.9 g	0 mg	37 mg	1.1 mg	0 mcg	0 mcg
18 g	16 g	0.1 mg	15.4 mg	0.2 mg	0 IU	0 mcg
12 g	10 g	0 mg	22 mg	0 mg	0 mcg	0 mcg
15 g	15 g	0 mg	13 mg	0 mg	0 mcg	0 mcg
27 g	23 g	0 mg	40 mg	0 mg	0 mcg	0 mcg
16 g	14 g	0 mg	11 mg	0 mg	0 mcg	0 mcg
14 g	8.2 g	0 mg	31 mg	0 mg	0 mcg	0 mcg
12 g	6.8 g	0 mg	47 mg	0.75 mg	0 mcg	0 mcg

Lemon	1 fruit	11.7	0 g	0.2 g	0.5 mg	0.2 g
Lime	1 fruit	11	0 g	0.2 g	0.9 mg	0.2 g
Mango	1 cup	107	0.36 g	1.6 g	3.3 mg	3.3 g
Oranges	1 large	87	0.21 g	1.9 g	0 mg	3.7 g
Passion fruit	1 fruit	17.5	0.1 g	0.4 g	5 mg	1.9 g
Peaches	1 fruit	61	0.35 g	1.6 g	0 mg	3.1 g
Pears	1 fruit	121	0.23 g	0 g	2.1 mg	6.3 g
Pineapple	1 cup	82.5	0.2 g	0.9 g	1.7 mg	2.3 g
Plums	1 fruit	31	0.22 g	0.67 g	0 mg	0.67 g
Pomegranate	1 fruit	105	0.51 g	1.5 g	4.6 mg	1.5 g
Raspberries	1 cup	64	1.2 g	1.2 g	1.2 mg	8.6 g
Strawberries	1 cup	48.6	0.5 g	1 g	1.5 mg	3 g
Tangerine	1 cup	103	0.6 g	1.6 g	3.9 mg	3.5 g
Watermelon	1 cup	46	0.17 g	1.5 g	1.5 mg	0 g

Grains

Food	Serving Size	Calories	Fat	Protein	Sodium	Fiber
Amaranth	¼ cup	182	3.2 g	7 g	10 mg	4.5 g
Bagel	1 bagel (3" diameter)	146	0.9 g	5.7 g	255 mg	1.3 g
Barley, flakes	1 cup	141	1.1 g	4 g	186 mg	3.4 g
Barley, pearled	¼ cup	176	0.56 g	5 g	4.5 mg	8 g
Buckwheat flour	¼ cup	101	0.9 g	3.9 g	3.3 mg	3 g
Buckwheat groats	1 cup	155	1 g	5.7 g	6.7 mg	4.5 g
Bulgur	1 cup	151	0.4 g	5.5 g	9.1 mg	9.1 g
Cornmeal	½ cup	251	1.4 g	5.5 g	2.1 mg	4.8 g
Couscous	1 cup cooked	175	0.17 g	6.3 g	7.8 mg	1.6 g
Couscous, whole wheat	¼ cup	173	1.5 g	7.5 g	0 mg	4.5 g
Cream of wheat	1 cup	31.5	0.6 g	4.4 g	364 mg	1.4 g
English muffin	1 muffin	140	1.1 g	5.4 g	248 mg	1.5 g
Flour tortilla	1 tortilla (51 grams)	146	3.1 g	4.4 g	249 mg	0 g

Carbohydrates	Sugar	Zinc	Calcium	Iron	Vitamin D	Vitamin B12
4.1 g	1.1 g	0 mg	3.3 mg	0 mg	0 mcg	0 mcg
3.7 g	0.7 g	0 mg	6.2 mg	0 mg	0 mcg	0 mcg
28 g	25 g	0 mg	16 mg	0 mg	0 mcg	0 mcg
22 g	17 g	0 mg	74 mg	0 mg	0 mcg	0 mcg
4.2 g	2 g	0 mg	2.2 mg	0.3 mg	0 mcg	0 mcg
16 g	13 g	0 mg	9.4 mg	0 mg	0 mcg	0 mcg
31 g	21 g	0 mg	19 mg	0 mg	0 mcg	0 mcg
21.6 g	16.3 g	0.2 mg	21.5 mg	0.5 mg	0 IU	0 mcg
7.3 g	6.7 g	0 mg	4 mg	0 mg	0 mcg	0 mcg
26 g	26 g	0 mg	4.6 mg	0 mg	0 mcg	0 mcg
15 g	4.9 g	0 mg	31 mg	1.2 mg	0 mcg	0 mcg
11.7 g	7.4 g	0.2 mg	24.3 mg	0.6 mg	0 IU	0 mcg
26 g	20.6 g	0.1 mg	72.2 mg	0.3 mg	0 mcg	0 mcg
12 g	9.2 g	0 mg	11 mg	0 mg	0 mcg	0 mcg

Carbohydrates	Sugar	Zinc	Calcium	Iron	Vitamin D	Vitamin B12
32 g	0 g	1.5 mg	75 mg	3.7 mg	0 mcg	0 mcg
29 g	2.9 g	1.1 mg	50.7 mg	3.4 mg	0 mcg	0 mcg
32 g	6.8 g	1.6 mg	15 mg	11 mg	27 mcg	2 mcg
39 g	0.5 g	1 mg	15 mg	1.5 mg	0 mcg	0 mcg
21 g	0.9 g	0.9 mg	12 mg	1.2 mg	0 mcg	0 mcg
34 g	1.5 g	1 mg	12 mg	1.3 mg	0 mcg	0 mcg
35 g	0 g	1.8 mg	18 mg	1.8 mg	0 mcg	0 mcg
53 g	0.68 g	0.68 mg	3.4 mg	2.7 mg	0 mcg	0 mcg
36 g	0 g	0 mg	13 mg	0 mg	0 mcg	0 mcg
36 g	0.8 g	0 mg	20 mg	1.82 mg	0 mcg	0 mcg
31.5 g	0.2 g	0.4 mg	154 mg	12 mg	0 mcg	0 mcg
27.4 g	1.8 g	0.7 mg	102 mg	2.4 mg	0 mcg	0 mcg
25.3 g	0 g	0 mg	97.4 mg	1 mg	0 mcg	0 mcg

Granola	⅓ cup	194	10 g	5.2 g	71.1 mg	3.7 g
Grits	1 cup	143	0.5 g	3.4 g	540 mg	0.7 g
Millet	¼ cup	189	2 g	5.5 g	2.5 mg	4.5 g
Oat bran	¼ cup	56	2 g	4 g	1 mg	3 g
Oat groats	¼ cup	110	2.5 g	7 g	0 mg	4 g
Oats, steel-cut	½ cup	152	2.7 g	6.6 g	0.78 mg	4.3 g
Pita	1 pita (6½" diameter)	165	0.7 g	5.5 g	322 mg	1.3 g
Polenta	½ cup	252	1.1 g	6 g	2.1 mg	5 g
Quinoa	1 cup	222	3.6 g	8.1 g	13 mg	5.2 g
Rice, brown	1 cup	216	1.8 g	5 g	9.8 mg	3.5 g
Rice cake	1 oz.	110	1.2 g	2 g	19.9 mg	1.2 g
Rice noodles	1 cup	192	0.4 g	1.6 g	33.4 mg	1.8 g
Rice, white	1 cup	169	0.3 g	3.5 g	8.7 mg	1.7 g
Rye	¼ cup	146	1.3 g	6.4 g	2.5 mg	6.4 g
Soba noodles	1 cup	113	0.1 g	5.8 g	68.4 mg	0 g
Spelt	1 cup cooked	246	1.6 g	10 g	9.7 mg	7.6 g
Spelt bread	1 slice	70	0 g	3 g	150 mg	2 g
Taco shell, hard	1 shell (5" diameter)	58.2	2.6 g	0.9 g	48.6 mg	0.6 g
Teff	½ cup uncooked	354	2.3 g	12.8 g	11.5 mg	7.7 g
Triticale	¼ cup	161	1 g	6.3 g	2.4 mg	0 g
Panfried polenta	1 oz.	101	1 g	2.3 g	9.8 mg	2 g
Pizza dough	2 oz.	120	1.1 g	4 g	240 mg	2 g
Popcorn	1 cup	30.6	0.3 g	1 g	0.3 mg	1.2 g
Vegetable pasta	½ cup	76	0.57 g	2.9 g	3.4 mg	0 g
Wheat berries	½ cup	151	1 g	6 g	0 mg	4 g
Whole grain bread	1 slice	69.1	1.1 g	3.5 g	110 mg	1.9 g
Whole grain cereal	¾ cup	100	0.5 g	2 g	190 mg	2.7 g
Whole-wheat pasta	½ cup	100	1.7 g	5 g	308 mg	2.5 g

23.2 g	7.7 g	1.2 mg	36.7 mg	1.4 mg	0 mcg	0 mcg
31.1 g	0.2 g	0.2 mg	7.3 mg	1.5 mg	0 mcg	0 mcg
37 g	0 g	1 mg	4 mg	1.5 mg	0 mcg	0 mcg
15 g	0 g	1 mg	13 mg	1 mg	0 mcg	0 mcg
27 g	1 g	0 mg	20 mg	0 mg	0 mcg	0 mcg
26 g	0 g	1.6 mg	21 mg	2 mg	0 mcg	0 mcg
33.4 g	0.8 g	0.5 mg	51.6 mg	1.6 mg	0 mcg	0 mcg
54 g	0.44 g	0.5 mg	3.4 mg	2.8 mg	0 mcg	0 mcg
39.4 g	0 g	2 mg	31.5 mg	2.8 mg	0 mcg	0 mcg
44.8 g	0.7 g	1.2 mg	19.5 mg	0.8 mg	0 mcg	0 mcg
22.7 g	0.2 g	0.8 mg	3.1 mg	0.4 mg	0 mcg	0 mcg
43.8 g	0 g	0.4 mg	7 mg	0.2 mg	0 mcg	0 mcg
36.7 g	0.1 g	0.7 mg	3.5 mg	0.2 mg	0 mcg	0 mcg
30 g	0.42 g	1.7 mg	14 mg	1.3 mg	0 mcg	0 mcg
24.4 g	0 g	0.1 mg	4.6 mg	0.5 mg	0 mcg	0 mcg
51 g	0 g	2.4 mg	19.4 mg	3.2 mg	0 mcg	0 mcg
16 g	2 g	0 mg	0 mg	0 mg	0 mcg	0 mcg
7.9 g	0.2 g	0.2 mg	12.6 mg	0.2 mg	0 mcg	0 mcg
70 g	1.8 g	3.5 mg	173 mg	7 mg	0 mcg	0 mcg
35 g	0 g	1.7 mg	18 mg	1.2 mg	0 mcg	0 mcg
21.5 g	0.2 g	0.5 mg	1.7 mg	1 mg	0 mcg	0 mcg
24 g	0 g	0 mg	0 mg	0 mg	0 mcg	0 mcg
6.2 g	0 g	0.3 mg	0.8 mg	0.2 mg	0 mcg	0 mcg
14 g	0 g	0.57 mg	10 mg	0.57 mg	0 mcg	0 mcg
29 g	0 g	5.6 mg	15 mg	7 mg	0 mcg	0 mcg
11.3 g	1.7 g	0.4 mg	26.6 mg	0.7 mg	0 mcg	0 mcg
23.2 g	5 g	15 mg	1,000 mg	18 mg	39.9 mcg	6 mcg
23 g	0 g	0.5 mg	14 mg	1.5 mg	0 mcg	0 mcg

Meat Replacements

Food	Serving Size	Calories	Fat	Protein	Sodium	Fiber
Black bean burger	1 patty	264	1 g	15 g	391 mg	9.7 g
Falafel	1 patty	57	3 g	2.3 g	50 mg	1 g
Ground beef substitute (sautéed)	½ cup	60	0.5 g	13 g	270 mg	3 g
Seitan	3 oz.	90	1 g	18 g	380 mg	1 g
Tempeh	½ cup	161	9.2 g	16 g	7.5 mg	0 g
Tofu, baked	½ cup	88.2	5.3 g	10.3 g	15.1 mg	1.1 g
Vegan sausage	1 patty	80	3 g	10 g	260 mg	1 g
Vegetarian chicken	3 oz.	120	5 g	9 g	210 mg	4 g
Vegetarian chicken patty burger	1 patty	140	5 g	8 g	590 mg	2 g
Veggie burger	1 patty	124	4.4 g	11 g	398 mg	3.4 g
Vegetarian hot dogs	1 link	80	2 g	11 g	390 mg	3 g
Vegetarian pepperoni	13 slices	50	1 g	9 g	240 mg	1 g

Nuts and Seeds

Food	Serving Size	Calories	Fat	Protein	Sodium	Fiber
Almond	1 oz.	161	13.8 g	5.9 g	0.3 mg	3.4 g
Brazil nuts	¼ cup	218	22 g	4.75 g	1 mg	2.5 g
Cashew	1 oz.	155	12.3 g	5.1 g	3.4 mg	0.9 g
Chestnuts, roasted	½ cup	175	1.6 g	2.1 g	1.4 mg	3.6 g
Chia seed	½ oz.	69	4.4 g	2.2 g	2.7 mg	5.3 g
Flaxseed	2 T.	104	8.2 g	3.5 g	5.9 mg	5.3 g
Hazelnut	¼ cup	180	18 g	4.3 g	0 mg	2.9 g
Macadamia nuts	¼ cup	239	25 g	3 g	2 mg	3 g
Nuts, mixed	1 oz.	172	15.7 g	4.3 g	85.7 mg	1.5 g
Peanuts, dry-roasted	1 oz.	164	13.9 g	6.6 g	1.7 mg	2.2 g
Peanuts, oil-roasted	1 oz.	168	14.7 g	7.8 g	89.6 mg	2.6 g
Pecans	1 oz.	193	20.2 g	2.6 g	0 mg	2.7 g
Pine nuts	¼ cup	190	17 g	8.3 g	1.2 mg	1.2 g
Pistachios	¼ cup	170	13 g	6.4 g	0.3 mg	3 g

Carbohydrates	Sugar	Zinc	Calcium	Iron	Vitamin D	Vitamin B$_{12}$
49 g	1.4 g	2.6 mg	79 mg	3.8 mg	0 mcg	0 mcg
5.4 g	0 g	0.26 mg	9.2 mg	0.58 mg	0 mcg	0 mcg
6 g	0 g	0 mg	60 mg	1.8 mg	0 IU	0 mcg
3 g	0 g	0 mg	0 mg	1 mg	0 IU	0 mcg
7.5 g	0 g	0.83 mg	93 mg	2.5 mg	0 mcg	0 mcg
2.1 g	0.8 g	1 mg	253 mg	2 mg	0 IU	0 mcg
3 g	1 g	0 mg	3 mg	1.44 mg	0 IU	2.1 mcg
11 g	0 g	0 mg	35 mg	15 mg	0 IU	0 mcg
16 g	1 g	0 mg	0 mg	0 mg	0 IU	0 mcg
10 g	0.7 g	0.9 mg	95.2 mg	1.7 mg	0 mcg	1.4 mcg
5 g	0 g	0 mg	2 mg	4 mg	0 mcg	0 mcg
2 g	0 g	0 mg	0 mg	0.36 mg	0 mcg	0 mcg

Carbohydrates	Sugar	Zinc	Calcium	Iron	Vitamin D	Vitamin B$_{12}$
6.1 g	1.1 g	0.9 mg	73.9 mg	1 mg	0 IU	0 mcg
4 g	0.77 g	1.35 mg	53.25 mg	0.8 mg	0 mcg	0 mcg
9.2 g	1.7 g	1.6 mg	10.4 mg	1.9 mg	0 IU	0 mcg
38 g	7.9 g	0.71 mg	21 mg	0.71 mg	0 mcg	0 mcg
6.2 g	0 g	0.49 mg	89 mg	0 mg	0 mcg	0 mcg
5.7 g	0.39 g	0.78 mg	50 mg	1.2 mg	0 mcg	0 mcg
4.9 g	1.1 g	0.57 mg	33 mg	1.4 mg	0 mcg	0 mcg
5 g	2 g	0 mg	28 mg	1 mg	0 mcg	0 mcg
6.2 g	1.2 g	1.3 mg	29.7 mg	0.7 mg	0 IU	0 mcg
6 g	1.2 g	0.9 mg	15.1 mg	0.6 mg	0 mcg	0 mcg
4.3 g	1.2 g	0.9 mg	17.1 mg	0.4 mg	0 IU	0 mcg
3.9 g	1.1 g	1.3 mg	19.6 mg	0.7 mg	0 IU	0 mcg
4.8 g	0 g	0 mg	8.3 mg	3.6 mg	0 mcg	0 mcg
8.5 g	2.4 g	0.61 mg	33 mg	1.2 mg	0 mcg	0 mcg

Food	Serving Size	Calories	Fat	Protein	Sodium	Fiber
Pumpkin seeds	¼ cup	185	16 g	8.6 g	6.2 mg	1.4 g
Soy nut	1 oz.	126	6.1 g	11.1 g	0.6 mg	2.3 g
Sunflower seeds	¼ cup	65	5.7 g	2.6 g	0.34 mg	1.3 g
Walnuts	1 oz.	185	18.4 g	4.3 g	0.6 mg	1.9 g

Vegetables

Food	Serving Size	Calories	Fat	Protein	Sodium	Fiber
Alfalfa sprouts	1 cup	10	0 g	1 g	2 mg	1 g
Artichokes	1 medium	60	0 g	4 g	114 mg	6.9 g
Asparagus	1 cup	27	0.15 g	2.7 g	2.7 mg	2.7 g
Asparagus, steamed	½ cup	19.8	0.2 g	2.2 g	12.6 mg	1.8 g
Beans, baked	½ cup	120	0.5 g	6 g	480 mg	6 g
Beans, black	1 cup canned	227	0.9 g	15.2 g	1.7 mg	15 g
Beans, butter	½ cup canned	110	0.5 g	6 g	420 mg	5 g
Beans, cannellini	½ cup canned	154	0.44 g	9.2 g	6.6 mg	6.6 g
Beans, fava	1 cup canned	182	0.57 g	13 g	375 mg	10 g
Beans, garbanzo	¾ cup canned	213	2 g	9 g	534 mg	7.1 g
Beans, kidney	1 cup canned, rinsed	210	2.6 g	13 g	759 mg	10 g
Beans, lima	¼ cup uncooked	151	0.45 g	9.4 g	8 mg	8.5 g
Beans, mung	¼ cup uncooked	180	0.6 g	12 g	7.8 mg	8.4 g
Beans, navy	½ cup canned	148	0.56 g	9.9 g	586 mg	6.7 g
Beans, pinto	1 cup cooked	205	2 g	12 g	23 mg	12 g
Beans, refried	1 cup	217	2.8 g	12.9 g	1,069 mg	12.1 g
Beans, yellow wax	1 cup	27	0.14 g	1.6 g	2.7 mg	1.8 g
Bean sprouts	1 cup	31	0 g	3 g	0 mg	2 g
Beets	1 cup	58	0.3 g	2.7 g	105 mg	4.1 g

6.2 g	0.34 g	2.4 mg	15 mg	5.1 mg	0 mcg	0 mcg
9.2 g	0 g	1.3 mg	39.2 mg	1.1 mg	0 mcg	0 mcg
2.2 g	0.34 g	0.57 mg	13 mg	0.8 mg	0 mcg	0 mcg
3.9 g	0.7 g	0.9 mg	27.7 mg	0.8 mg	0 IU	0 mcg

Carbohydrates	Sugar	Zinc	Calcium	Iron	Vitamin D	Vitamin B$_{12}$
1 g	0 g	0 mg	11 mg	0 mg	0 mcg	0 mcg
13 g	0 g	0.63 mg	56 mg	1.6 mg	0 mcg	0 mcg
5.3 g	2.7 g	1.3 mg	32 mg	2.7 mg	0 mcg	0 mcg
3.7 g	1.2 g	0.5 mg	20.7 mg	0.8 mg	0 mcg	0 mcg
24 g	9 g	2.1 mg	40 mg	2.7 mg	0 IU	0 mcg
40.8 g	0 g	1.9 mg	46.4 mg	3.6 mg	0 IU	0 mcg
19 g	0 g	0 mg	60 mg	1.79 mg	0 mcg	0 mcg
29 g	0 g	1.3 mg	96 mg	3.9 mg	0 mcg	0 mcg
31 g	0 g	2.6 mg	67 mg	2.6 mg	0 mcg	0 mcg
41 g	0 g	1.8 mg	57 mg	1.8 mg	0 mcg	0 mcg
38 g	5.1 g	0 mg	87 mg	2.6 mg	0 mcg	0 mcg
28 g	4 g	1.3 mg	36 mg	3.6 mg	0 mcg	0 mcg
32 g	3.4 g	1.4 mg	68 mg	3.5 mg	0 mcg	0 mcg
27 g	0.37 g	1 mg	62 mg	2.4 mg	0 mcg	0 mcg
36 g	0 g	2.4 mg	102 mg	2.4 mg	0 mcg	0 mcg
36.3 g	1.1 g	1.5 mg	78.6 mg	4 mg	0 IU	0 mcg
6.1 g	1.3 g	0.39 mg	35 mg	1.2 mg	0 mcg	0 mcg
6 g	4 g	0 mg	0 mg	0 mg	0 IU	0 mcg
14 g	9.5 g	0 mg	22 mg	1.4 mg	0 mcg	0 mcg

Beet greens	1 cup	8	0 g	0.77 g	87 mg	1.5 g
Bok choy	1 cup	20	0 g	2 g	90 mg	2 g
Broccoli rabe	1 cup, chopped	8.8	0.2 g	1.3 g	13.2 mg	1.1 g
Broccoli, raw	1 cup	30.9	0.3 g	2.6 g	30 mg	2.4 g
Broccoli, steamed	1 stalk, 1 cup	49	0.6 g	3.3 g	57.4 mg	4.6 g
Brussels sprouts	1 cup	61	1 g	4 g	33 mg	4 g
Cabbage	1 cup	22	0.1 g	0.91 g	16 mg	1.8 g
Carrots	1 cup	52.5	0.3 g	1.2 g	88.3 mg	3.6 g
Carrots, baby	3 oz.	29.8	0.1 g	0.5 g	66.3 mg	2.5 g
Cauliflower	1 cup	25	0.11 g	2 g	30 mg	3 g
Celery	1 cup	14	0.22 g	1 g	81 mg	2 g
Collard greens	1 cup	11	0.16 g	0.71 g	7.1 mg	1.4 g
Corn on the cob	1 ear	155	3.4 g	4.5 g	29.2 mg	0 g
Cucumber	1 cucumber	45.1	0.3 g	2 g	6 mg	1.5 g
Edamame	1 cup	189	8.1 g	16.9 g	9.3 mg	8.1 g
Eggplant	1 cup	32.7	0.2 g	0.8 g	237 mg	2.5 g
Endives	2 cups	17	0.22 g	1 g	22 mg	3 g
Kale	1 cup	33	0.67 g	2 g	29 mg	1.3 g
Kohlrabi	1 cup	36	0.15 g	2.7 g	27 mg	5.4 g
Leeks	1 cup	55	0.3 g	1.8 g	18 mg	1.8 g
Lentils	¼ cup uncooked	170	0.53 g	13 g	2.9 mg	15 g
Lettuce, iceberg	1 cup	10.1	0.1 g	0.6 g	7.2 mg	0.9 g
Lettuce, romaine	1 cup	8	0.1 g	0.6 g	3.8 mg	1 g
Mushrooms, portabello	1 medium	29	0.25 g	3.4 g	6.8 mg	2.3 g
Mushrooms, shiitake	1 cup	81	0.32 g	2.9 g	5.8 mg	2.9 g
Mushrooms, white button	1 cup	16	0.24 g	2.1 g	3.6 mg	0.71 g
Olives, green	1 oz.	40.6	4.3 g	0.3 g	436 mg	0.9 g
Okra	1 cup	31	0.11 g	2 g	8 mg	3 g
Onion, boiled pearl	1 cup	43	0 g	0 g	0 mg	0 g

1.5 g	0.38 g	0 mg	45 mg	1.2 mg	0 mcg	0 mcg
4 g	0 g	4.3 mg	32 mg	1.1 mg	0 mcg	0 mcg
1.2 g	0.2 g	0.3 mg	43.2 mg	0.9 mg	0 mcg	0 mcg
6 g	1.5 g	0.4 mg	42.8 mg	0.7 mg	0 mcg	0 mcg
10.1 g	1.9 g	0.6 mg	56 mg	0.9 mg	0 IU	0 mcg
14 g	0 g	0 mg	56 mg	2 mg	0 mcg	0 mcg
5.5 g	3.6 g	0 mg	43 mg	0.91 mg	0 mcg	0 mcg
12.3 g	6.1 g	0.3 mg	42.4 mg	0.4 mg	0 mcg	0 mcg
7 g	4 g	0.1 mg	27.2 mg	0.8 mg	0 IU	0 mcg
5 g	2 g	0 mg	22 mg	0 mg	0 mcg	0 mcg
3 g	2 g	0 mg	40 mg	0 mg	0 mcg	0 mcg
2.1 g	0 g	0 mg	52 mg	0 mg	0 mcg	0 mcg
31.9 g	0 g	0.9 mg	4.4 mg	0.9 mg	0 IU	0 mcg
10.9 g	5 g	0.6 mg	48.2 mg	0.8 mg	0 IU	0 mcg
15.8 g	3.4 g	2.1 mg	97.6 mg	3.5 mg	0 IU	0 mcg
8.1 g	3.2 g	0.1 mg	5.9 mg	0.2 mg	0 IU	0 mcg
3 g	0 g	1 mg	52 mg	1 mg	0 mcg	0 mcg
6.7 g	0 g	0 mg	90 mg	1.3 mg	0 mcg	0 mcg
8.1 g	4.1 g	0 mg	32 mg	0 mg	0 mcg	0 mcg
13 g	3.6 g	0 mg	54 mg	1.8 mg	0 mcg	0 mcg
29 g	0.96 g	2.4 mg	27 mg	3.8 mg	0 mcg	0 mcg
2.3 g	1.4 g	0.1 mg	13 mg	0.3 mg	0 IU	0 mcg
1.5 g	0.6 g	0.1 mg	15.5 mg	0.5 mg	0 IU	0 mcg
5.7 g	2.3 g	1.1 mg	9.1 mg	1.1 mg	0 mcg	0 mcg
20 g	5.8 g	1.4 mg	4.3 mg	0 mg	0 mcg	0 mcg
2.1 g	1.4 g	0.71 mg	2.1 mg	0.71 mg	0 mcg	0 mcg
1.1 g	0.2 g	0 mg	14.6 mg	0.1 mg	0 IU	0 mcg
7 g	1 g	1 mg	81 mg	1 mg	0 mcg	0 mcg
1 g	0 g	0 mg	3.1 mg	0 mg	0 mcg	0 mcg

Onion, red	1 onion	42	0 g	0 g	0 mg	0 g
Parsnips	1 cup	100	0.44 g	1.3 g	13 mg	6.7 g
Peas	1 cup	117	0.64 g	7.2 g	7.2 mg	7.2 g
Peas, black-eyed	1 cup canned	199	3.8 g	6.6 g	839 mg	7.9 g
Pepper, green bell	1 cup	29.8	0.3 g	1.3 g	4.5 mg	2.5 g
Pepper, jalapeño	1 pepper	4	0.14 g	0.14 g	0.14 mg	0.42 g
Pepper, roasted red bell	1 oz.	9.3	0 g	0 g	112 mg	0.9 g
Pepper, yellow bell	1 pepper	32	0 g	1 g	2 mg	2 g
Potatoes	1 small (138 grams)	128	0.2 g	3.5 g	13.8 mg	3 g
Pumpkin	1 cup	30	0.13 g	1.2 g	1.2 mg	1.2 g
Rutabaga	1 cup	51	0.31 g	1.4 g	28 mg	4.2 g
Spinach	1 cup	6.9	0.1 g	0.9 g	23.7 mg	0.7 g
Spinach, steamed	1 cup	41.4	0.5 g	5.3 g	126 mg	4.3 g
Squash, acorn	1 cup	56	0.16 g	1.4 g	4.2 mg	2.8 g
Squash, oven-roasted butternut	1 cup	82	0.2 g	1.8 g	8.2 mg	0 g
Squash, spaghetti	1 cup	41.9	0.4 g	1 g	27.9 mg	2.2 g
Squash, summer	1 cup	18	0.25 g	1.1 g	2.3 mg	1.1 g
Sweet potato	1 small (60 grams)	54	0.1 g	1.2 g	21.6 mg	2 g
Swiss chard	1 cup	7	0 g	0.71 g	76 mg	0.71 g
Tomato	1 medium	22.1	0.2 g	1.1 g	6.2 mg	1.5 g
Turnips	1 large	51	0.2 g	1.8 g	122 mg	3.6 g
Water chestnuts	¼ cup	30	0 g	0.31 g	4.3 mg	0.93 g
Watercress	¼ cup	1	0 g	0.17 g	3.5 mg	0 g
Yams	1 cup	176	0.33 g	3 g	13 mg	6 g
Zucchini	1 cup	19.8	0.2 g	1.5 g	12.4 mg	1.4 g
Zucchini, sautéed	1 cup	28.8	0.1 g	1.2 g	5.4 mg	2.5 g

1 g	0 g	0 mg	3 mg	1.2 mg	0 mcg	0 mcg
24 g	6.7 g	1.3 mg	48 mg	1.3 mg	0 mcg	0 mcg
20 g	8.7 g	1.4 mg	36 mg	1.4 mg	0 mcg	0 mcg
40 g	0 g	2.5 mg	41 mg	3.4 mg	0 mcg	0 mcg
6.9 g	3.6 g	0.2 mg	14.9 mg	0.5 mg	0 mcg	0 mcg
0.85 g	0.42 g	0 mg	1.4 mg	0.14 mg	0 mcg	0 mcg
3.7 g	0.9 g	0 mg	0 mg	1 mg	0 IU	0 mcg
8 g	0 g	0 mg	11 mg	1 mg	0 mcg	0 mcg
29.2 g	1.6 g	0.5 mg	20.7 mg	1.5 mg	0 IU	0 mcg
8.1 g	1.2 g	0 mg	24 mg	1.2 mg	0 mcg	0 mcg
11 g	8.5 g	0 mg	66 mg	1.4 mg	0 mcg	0 mcg
1.1 g	0.1 g	0.2 mg	29.7 mg	0.8 mg	0 IU	0 mcg
6.7 g	0.8 g	1.4 mg	245 mg	6.4 mg	0 IU	0 mcg
14 g	0 g	0 mg	46 mg	1.4 mg	0 mcg	0 mcg
21.5 g	4 g	0.3 mg	84 mg	1.2 mg	0 IU	0 mcg
10 g	3.9 g	0.3 mg	32.6 mg	0.5 mg	0 mcg	0 mcg
3.4 g	2.3 g	0 mg	17 mg	0 mg	0 mcg	0 mcg
12.4 g	3.9 g	0.2 mg	22.8 mg	0.4 mg	0 IU	0 mcg
1.4 g	0.36 g	0 mg	18 mg	0.71 mg	0 mcg	0 mcg
4.8 g	3.2 g	0.2 mg	12.3 mg	0.3 mg	0 IU	0 mcg
11 g	7.3 g	0 mg	55 mg	0 mg	0 mcg	0 mcg
7.4 g	1.5 g	0.31 mg	3.4 mg	0 mg	0 mcg	0 mcg
0 g	0 g	0 mg	10 mg	0 mg	0 mcg	0 mcg
42 g	1.5 g	0 mg	25 mg	1.5 mg	0 mcg	0 mcg
4.2 g	2.1 g	0.4 mg	18.6 mg	0.4 mg	0 mcg	0 mcg
7.1 g	3 g	0.3 mg	23.4 mg	0.6 mg	0 IU	0 mcg

US/Metric Conversion Chart

VOLUME CONVERSIONS

US Volume Measure	Metric Equivalent
⅛ teaspoon	0.5 milliliter
¼ teaspoon	1 milliliter
½ teaspoon	2 milliliters
1 teaspoon	5 milliliters
½ tablespoon	7 milliliters
1 tablespoon (3 teaspoons)	15 milliliters
2 tablespoons (1 fluid ounce)	30 milliliters
¼ cup (4 tablespoons)	60 milliliters
⅓ cup	90 milliliters
½ cup (4 fluid ounces)	125 milliliters
⅔ cup	160 milliliters
¾ cup (6 fluid ounces)	180 milliliters
1 cup (16 tablespoons)	250 milliliters
1 pint (2 cups)	500 milliliters
1 quart (4 cups)	1 liter (about)

WEIGHT CONVERSIONS

US Weight Measure	Metric Equivalent
½ ounce	15 grams
1 ounce	30 grams
2 ounces	60 grams
3 ounces	85 grams
¼ pound (4 ounces)	115 grams
½ pound (8 ounces)	225 grams
¾ pound (12 ounces)	340 grams
1 pound (16 ounces)	454 grams

OVEN TEMPERATURE CONVERSIONS

Degrees Fahrenheit	Degrees Celsius
200 degrees F	95 degrees C
250 degrees F	120 degrees C
275 degrees F	135 degrees C
300 degrees F	150 degrees C
325 degrees F	160 degrees C
350 degrees F	180 degrees C
375 degrees F	190 degrees C
400 degrees F	205 degrees C
425 degrees F	220 degrees C
450 degrees F	230 degrees C

BAKING PAN SIZES

American	Metric
8 × 1½ inch round baking pan	20 × 4 cm cake tin
9 × 1½ inch round baking pan	23 × 3.5 cm cake tin
11 × 7 × 1½ inch baking pan	28 × 18 × 4 cm baking tin
13 × 9 × 2 inch baking pan	30 × 20 × 5 cm baking tin
2 quart rectangular baking dish	30 × 20 × 3 cm baking tin
15 × 10 × 2 inch baking pan	30 × 25 × 2 cm baking tin (Swiss roll tin)
9 inch pie plate	22 × 4 or 23 × 4 cm pie plate
7 or 8 inch springform pan	18 or 20 cm springform or loose bottom cake tin
9 × 5 × 3 inch loaf pan	23 × 13 × 7 cm or 2 lb narrow loaf or pâté tin
1½ quart casserole	1.5 liter casserole
2 quart casserole	2 liter casserole

Index